YOU CAN'T FIX THEM—BECAUSE THEY'RE NOT BROKEN

A Sustainability Guide for Tired Helpers & Healers

Jo Eckler, Psy.D., RYT

Spiral Staircase Publishing

AUSTIN, TEXAS

Bulk discounts available for educational and training programs.

Jo Eckler c/o Spiral Staircase Publishing
3005 S. Lamar Blvd., Ste D-109 #214
Austin, TX 78704
www.spiralstaircasepublishing.com
www.joeckler.com

Publisher's Note: This work is not a substitute for professional psychotherapy or other mental health treatment. Using the techniques in this book does not guarantee any particular outcome, income, or business results.

Book Layout © 2017 BookDesignTemplates.com

Book Cover design and artwork by Amrit Elise Mayton © 2021 Jo Eckler

Author Photo by Loveolution Photography © 2020, used with permission

You can't fix them—because they're not broken: A sustainability guide for tired helpers and healers/Jo Eckler. -- 1st ed. Paperback.
ISBN 978-1-7346659-2-5

To all my teachers along the way.

.

CONTENTS

Why You're Here

You chose to become a healer, a helper because the world is full of pain. You might even have experienced some of (or a lot of) that pain yourself. Your heart aches for neglected children, for dying ecosystems, for the sick, the wounded, the repressed people wandering around lost and lonely. You can see all this, and naturally you were moved to do something about it.

Because you could see something else. You could see hope. Potential. The little light inside each living creature that could grow and glow if given the right nourishment and care.

So you set out on your mission. You collected tools. Sat through trainings. Devoured books and videos and lectures and certificates. You devoted tons of time, money, energy, brainpower, and love to learning your healing modality. You spent hours picking out the right supplies and accessories to create peaceful, safe spaces. Creating materials to give to your clients, maybe handouts, maybe essential oil blends, ordering herbs or choosing crystals.

Thus you began your journey as a healer, a helper. It felt right. It felt aligned and good and like you were finally doing what you came to this planet to do. You met your first clients with a mixture of excitement, wonder, and gratitude (perhaps with a dash of impostor syndrome). They thanked you; you saw some results. And it was awesome.

Like anything, the newness wore off, and it got less exciting and amazing that clients came to see you. But your confidence grew. You answered questions more smoothly, and you sharpened your sense of who was going to benefit from what type of help. Your early clients sent people your way. You'd found a rhythm. And it was pretty darn good.

Until it wasn't. Until a client came along that you couldn't seem to help, or who needed so much more from you than you could give. You might have taken on some of their despair or worry, or been shaken deeply by a painful memory that they shared with you. Or you started feeling bored. Maybe it got harder to get out of bed, or you looked at your schedule with dread, feeling trapped. You might even have had moments of resentment or bitterness towards a client as they talked about a lifestyle that you couldn't access or self-care that you hadn't been allowing yourself.

Your body may have gotten involved, developing aches, pains, and illnesses. Headaches, digestive problems, unsettled sleep, fatigue...all kinds of rebellion on the physical level. All signals that something has gone awry. The health issues might even have been enough to convince you to take time off or leave the healing profession altogether.

And now here you are, so far from that initial enthusiasm and openness with which you met your first clients. You might be feeling discouraged, despondent, disillusioned, perhaps a little desperate. You might even be ready to quit--if you haven't already.

And now here I am, having been a professional healer and helper myself for almost 20 years (and many more as an amateur before that), offering you the tools and information that I wish I'd had much earlier in my own journey. Here I am to tell you that there is hope for a more sustainable healing profession. There is hope for being a healthier helper, whether it's with people in your life or clients on your caseload.

My question to you is: Are you willing?

Are you willing to step back from your knowledgeable, expert place and shift into curiosity? Are you willing to try something new, even if you're not good at it right away? Are you willing to look deeply into the patterns and practices in your life and consider whether they're still serving you?

If you're not, then tuck this book away for a while or pass it along to a friend who can use it. It's okay. We're all ready at different times.

If you are willing, then let's begin right away. No reason you should suffer any longer than need be!

Allow yourself to shift into a place of not knowing. Of not having to facilitate anything, not having to monitor or know the next step or plan. You can simply be in student mode for now, receiving.

And what will you receive, you ask?

In the next chapters, I'll walk you through important areas to consider as a healer and helper. Each chapter will introduce a concept, give you practical tools for implementing that tool in your life, and provide exercises so you can practice them. These strategies combine professional and personal experience as well as scientific research. They're the same things I've taught the clinicians I've supervised and clients I've coached, and I've seen the difference they can make. Plus, I

4 · YOU CAN'T FIX THEM

know you're tired, overwhelmed, and busy, so I try to make these ideas as clear and simple for you as possible.

Sound good?

Here's your first exercise.

Inhale. Exhale long and slow out through the mouth. Take your time. Inhale. Exhale in a big, loud sigh. One more inhale. One more sigh.

Now take no more than 10 minutes and write your future self a letter about why you want to try using this book. Write about how you're feeling now. How you hope to feel. How making changes will affect other areas of your life. All of it. If you can write by hand, great. If you can't, that's totally fine. Feel free to type or make a voice recording instead. If you're more visual, then you can create a collage or other artwork that reminds you of where you are now, why you crave a change, and what you hope to see on the other side. Keep this reminder so you can return to it as needed!

(I use this exercise with all my clients, by the way. There's a messy middle in any change process, and it's helpful to refer back to our initial motivation for getting into it in the first place.)

1. What I've Learned the Hard Way

1.1 Content Warning

Before we go any farther, I want to let you know that this book does mention some of the painful and disturbing things that can happen in life. I only do so when necessary, and I try to avoid getting into graphic detail. Still, it's there.

Just like it'll show up when we meet with our clients. No matter what type of healing or helping work you do, at some point someone is going to tell you something that disturbs you.

When this happens with this book, you have a few options. You can:

1. Stop reading and never come back. Which is totally okay. There are other books out there.

2. Take a break, do a little grounding and self-care, then come back when you feel ready.

3. Use your reactions as a chance to practice the tools in this book.

4. Do something else entirely.
5. All of the above.

No judgment here, whatever you decide. If you're still willing and ready, let's get started so you can feel more prepared to help both yourself and your clients.

My career as a helper started in middle school. Seriously. And maybe yours did too, or even earlier. I was literally fielding suicide crisis calls in eighth grade, so often that my parents would just nod and excuse me from the table when I answered the dial and got that worried look on my face. I'd head down the hall to plop down on my bed and pick up the receiver and try to talk my friend into putting down the bleach bottle or pocketknife or whatever, trying to remind them of reasons to stick around and discover if things improve.

And it just kept going from there. I've always been that person. You know, the one at parties off in the corner listening to someone pouring out their heartbreak or fears. While at a bus stop, a fellow traveler would sit down next to me, and before the bus arrived, I would know all about their recent cancer diagnosis and childhood trauma. In college, my dorm room phone would wake me at all hours and I'd sleepily mumble reassuring words, hoping they'd do the trick.

It just kept going. And going. I felt important and special. Honored that people would entrust me with such serious issues before I was even old enough to buy a beer. Since I didn't feel awesome about myself in the first place, having this helper role reassured me that at least I was worth something to someone, that I could earn the right to exist with my sympathetic ear and hours of time. Losing myself in other people's problems was also a handy way to avoid looking at my own, and their needs were a good excuse for skipping out on my self-care. How could I possibly go work out when so-and-so was so upset about their grades/relationship/etc.?

I bet you can guess where this is going.

My attention and giving to others grew and grew and grew. My attention and giving to myself shrank and shrank and shrank.

And then it all exploded.

I was outside my dorm sitting on the sun-warmed concrete wall one afternoon, smoking a cigarette (yeah, the self-care wasn't great back then, remember?) after an extra-busy time of emotionally supporting friends and kinda-friends. I said to myself: "If one more goddamm person asks me for one more goddamm thing, I'm going to fucking lose it."

A passerby asked to bum a cigarette.

I melted down. Internally, of course. I didn't want to cause anyone any inconvenience. Even my breakdowns were polite.

And the next day I was at the front desk of the university counseling center.

The things I learned in therapy got me out of that vicious cycle of fury and resentment, but not far enough. Becoming a psychologist presented me with even tougher challenges, especially since I was focusing on helping trauma survivors like myself. It felt so good to be trusted, to be helpful, to be able to offer some techniques. At the same time, I quickly became overwhelmed and exhausted. One of the breaking points this time? When I actually dreamed one of my client's nightmares. It wasn't my nightmare or traumatic experience—it was a terrifying event she had shared in an intense session earlier that week. (If you're wondering, yes, that is definitely a sign that something has to change!)

1.2 How I Learned This Stuff

Therapy was probably one of the best things I ever did for myself. Besides processing piles of intense trauma, I also learned what healthy boundaries actually look like. My therapists have helped me see how helpful balance can be and that I can't (and don't have to!) be anyone's 24-hour crisis hotline. There are real crisis hotlines that have trained and paid staff who can do that—maybe you even work for one.

I did not learn it all before being handed my bachelor's degree, that's for sure. Years of life experience, professional training as I earned my doctorate in clinical psychology, yoga teacher trainings, learning how to do energy work, becoming a hospice volunteer, having cats, having partners, my own therapy and research, being a clinical supervisor, and working in multiple mental health settings have all taught me what to do—and not to do—when helping others. I've also learned vicariously by watching colleagues who burned out and those who carefully tended to their own health.

I'd love for you to be the latter. The ones who learned ways to make the work they love sustainable. The ones who shared their gifts with others while living fulfilling and enjoyable lives.

The other nifty bit is that as healers and helpers, whatever we learn is information that might be useful for a client down the road. Nothing is wasted. So if you can't do it for yourself right now, do it for those clients. Do it for your colleagues and trainees who need your example to give them permission for their own self-care. Do it for your loved ones who worry when they see you exhausted and snippy. And do it for your future self.

Merriam-Webster's definition of sustainable

1: capable of being sustained

2a: of, relating to, or being a method of harvesting or using a resource so that the resource is not depleted or permanently damaged; sustainable techniques; sustainable agriculture

b: of or relating to a lifestyle involving the use of sustainable methods; sustainable society

1.3 Using This Book

Consider this book your fellow traveler as you do your healing and helping work. It can be a colleague to turn to when you're feeling overwhelmed or stuck. It can serve as inspiration for ways to help your clients. And it can be a source of strength and encouragement in your personal life.

My previous book, *I Can't Fix You—Because You're Not Broken: The Eight Keys to Freeing Yourself From Painful Thoughts and Feelings*, also based in the principles of Acceptance and Commitment Therapy, makes an excellent companion to this book. If you like, you can assign your clients chapters to read and then discuss them together. You'll notice that some concepts are similar, although this book offers more in-depth explanations of how to use them with other people's thoughts and feelings, not just your own. This book will also cover practical topics unique to serving in a helping profession, such as how to handle systemic issues that arise in agencies and private practice.

Go through this book at a pace that suits you. Come back to it as many times as you like. These strategies and concepts are here to support you while you do the work of supporting others.

1.4 Why I Wrote This

I got lucky with graduate school. My program gave me five years of space, time, supervision, and education not just on techniques to help people (although I got plenty of those) but on "the music behind the words," the process of healing and what can arise in a healing relationship. My sessions were often recorded, and my supervisors would give me feedback based on what they observed. I know that length and depth of training is rare, even for some types of counselors. As I sat in yoga teacher trainings and energy work apprenticeships and learned to play the gong and so on, I could see how attention to these aspects of helping work was limited, sometimes simply because of time constraints. I couldn't help but compare it to the depth of training that I as a psychologist was expected to give the psychology practicum students and interns I supervised.

Many talented helpers have learned these things in their own way over time. I definitely do not want to dismiss anyone's skills and gifts! You might already know everything in this book. (In that case, gift it to a newly graduated helper or use it for kindling or something.) Still, just in case, I wanted to put together what I've learned so far in hopes of saving you some time and heartache. Even though I had extensive train-ing, there is so much that I wish someone had told me early in my career. So I'll do what I can to share that information with you.

2. Burnout and Compassion Fatigue

2.1 What They Are and How to Recognize Them

Ever reached a point where you felt like you were working all the time, devoting all your energy to it, yet getting very little done? Where no matter how many breaks you took or "fun" activities you did, everything felt blah? And nothing was recharging you--not coffee, not sleeping all weekend, not a beautiful day?

That's probably burnout.

And those times when you felt unmoved by a tragic story or thought that your clients (and maybe even your friends) were whining over petty issues?

Probably compassion fatigue.

"Fuck 'em," said Ford, slumping on the bed. "You can't care about every damn thing."

- Douglas Adams, Mostly Harmless

Burnout and compassion fatigue like to travel together, which makes for double trouble. So here you are feeling like an engine with a broken alternator, with a battery that nothing will recharge, and the world is suddenly full of people making big deals out of nothing. You're too tired to care. You've heard too many terrible stories. If you deal with the same problems regularly, you might be a little bored and could even find yourself mixing up clients' stories.

We healers and helpers don't like to talk about these things, especially if it seems like all our colleagues are managing just fine, walking around all fulfilled by their work and saving the world and shit. That unspoken pressure to "be grateful that you get to do such important work" and comments like "it must feel great to help people every day" can push us deeper and deeper into silence and shame.

We also worry that if we mention our slips and cynicism, we'll risk being considered incompetent. That can stir up fears for our licenses, our referral base, and our professional reputation. So more silence. More shame.

And what does that shame do? Keeps us isolated. Puts us into flight/flight/freeze mode. Exhausts us and drains our hope. Disconnects us from others when what we need most is empathy, validation of our struggles, and a non-judgmental ear.

I'll get real with you. If we stay stuck in shame and don't know ways to recognize and get out of it, it is destructive. This is where people leave the field, doctors lose licenses for substance abuse, helpers get in trouble for crossing boundaries, healers develop health consequences from overwork, and sometimes, tragically, helpers might even decide to end their own lives. Shame will devour us and munch on our life as we know it for dessert.

So, to recap. Burnout and compassion fatigue are common occupational hazards of any helping work. They're going to happen, just like an athlete will experience injuries during their career. These states of being are hard enough to deal with on their own, but if we believe they mean we are inferior or screwed up somehow, then watch out for shame joining the party. And shame has a scorched earth policy if allowed to grow unchecked.

Dr. Brené Brown gives us hope, however, with her reminder that: "If we can share our story with someone who responds with empathy and understanding, shame can't survive."

This book isn't just a list of tools for your toolbox. It's also me sharing what I've learned (the hard way) over the years and to offer you empathy and understanding. If you get nothing else out of it, I hope you leave with this: You're not the only one. You're not broken. You're just a human being doing really hard work for yourself and others.

Exercise:

What are your own warning signs of burnout and compassion fatigue?

Identify one safe person to talk to about your struggles. If you can't think of one, where are some places you could look for someone?

2.2 Risk Factors and Causes

Burnout can happen to anyone in any situation. However, the following factors make burnout more likely. How many are present in your current environment?

➢ More demand than resources.

➢ A group culture that considers expressions of anything except positivity to be "whining" or weakness.

➢ Unrealistic expectations, especially when coupled with negative consequences for not meeting them, and even more so when factors beyond your control make it impossible to meet those expectations.

➢ A lack of relationships and activities that are unrelated to the helping work.

➢ Difficulty asking for and accepting help.

➢ Situations where basic physical and safety needs are not being met (such as limited time for breaks or access to food and water, having to do home visits to challenging clients alone, long hours that impact ability to get adequate sleep, insufficient income creating worries about bills and finances).

➢ Personal worth being tied up in how hard you work and how many hours you work.

➢ History of your own unaddressed or processed issues, like trauma.

➢ A group culture that measures your value by what you can produce and/or how much you sacrifice.

If many of these sound familiar, you are likely at high risk for burnout. This doesn't mean you're doomed! This list is more like those yellow caution signs alongside the road warning you to be watchful and to up your sustainability game.

Exercise:

How many of the risk factors mentioned here are present in your current environment? Are there any you can change?

2.3 Abusive Workplaces

There's stress. There's burnout. And then there's bullying and abuse. The most important thing to remember if you are in an abusive situation is that the abuse is **not your fault**. There's no amount of deep breathing or time management that can change the fact that you're in an abusive situation--your primary task in that situation is to survive until you can figure out a safe way to leave. That's it. You can save the fancy stuff until you're in a safer place. You can even put this book aside until you're in a safer place.

All workers need to be aware of when a demanding work situation crosses the line into an abusive one. Since many of us healers and helpers feel called to our professions because we bear our own wounds, we run the additional risk of being retraumatized or triggered in our work situations, sometimes without realizing it.

Abuse can happen anytime to anyone. Here are some times when it might be particularly likely (for more details, see Feijó et al., 2019):

➢ During training or your first job, since you have no basis for comparison.

➢ When work roles and duties are unclear.

➢ High demands and workload.

➢ When you are isolated, the only one of your demographic, or lowest in status.

➢ Situations where an abusive higher-up engages in wrong-doing and they sense you are an ethical truth-teller.

➢ Historically overly demanding and authoritarian situations, such as during some medical school training, where the belief is that their training was abusive and demanding so yours should be too.

➢ Work situations where there are (or appear to be) few other options as far as places to train or work.

We can get used to anything when we've been taught to expect that a helping role will take everything we have to give. Abusive workplaces will gaslight you into thinking that you are selfish if you don't do everything they demand of you, no matter how excessive or unreasonable. Miserable martyrs are celebrated, and people trying to meet their basic needs are painted as self-indulgent.

Over time, these situations can wear you down and have you believing that you are inadequate and incompetent. Much like in an abusive romantic relationship, you can start believing that no other job would have you and that you're lucky that your current one tolerates you. You believe that you deserve this treatment because you are such a burden. Between the unreasonable workload and the emotional abuse, you can feel like changing jobs or career paths is impossible. You're too exhausted. It doesn't help that right when you're thinking seriously about leaving or standing up for yourself, the abusive person might become unusually sweet and generous, making you feel ungrateful and doubting your negative experiences. It can seem like every job will have the same terrible environment, that this is just how work is for everyone.

So here's your reminder that this is not true. There are workplaces that respect their staff. That allow you to take a day off without a huge guilt trip. That give you time to get a drink of water, to go to the bathroom, to eat lunch. Some will even invest in your professional development and encourage you to try new roles and skills. You don't have to leave every meeting feeling like you're a pitiful loser.

While you're still in the situation, stay connected with the people in your life who see your skills and potential. Let them remind you you're not as awful as your boss says, that you deserve to be treated like a human being. They can serve as your reality check and antidote to any gaslighting or manipulation that might be happening.

If you decide you want to leave the situation, ask those friends to help you make a thoughtful plan. In the meantime, many experts recommend you document the abusive behaviors, including date, time, any witnesses, and whatever specifics you can add. It's probably best to do this somewhere the abusive person can't access it, such as a personal notebook or in your personal email.

Whenever you do leave, as hard as it may be, taking the high road and leaving in a professional way will likely serve you better in the long run and deprives them of ammunition against you. Once you go, recognize that there will be a period of recovery. Depending on how you're feeling, therapy might be a good idea to help you process your experience and rebuild your faith in yourself.

2.4 How to Recover

The thing with burnout is, you can't go after it with the same frantic effort and hard work that got you burned out in the first place. Burnout requires an entirely different approach. You have to go into what will feel like slow-motion. Your mind might even label it as "lazy" or "slacking." A burned-out healer needs the same level of gentle, attentive holding as if you were carrying a thin, fine porcelain cup full of hot Earl Grey tea across the floor of a bouncy castle.

For many of us high achievers, the instinctive impulse is to do more. You might be tempted to go read everything there is to know about burnout, to go to three yoga classes a day, do an hour of meditation, completely change your diet and cook everything from scratch...stop! *You can't get out of overdoing it by overdoing it.*

For fast-acting relief, try slowing down.

-Lily Tomlin

Burnout needs space and rest. Staring out the window for a while is fine. Dozing on the couch is fine. Gentle movement that you enjoy is fine. Savoring delicious food is fine. Unscheduled hours are wonderful.

When your nervous system is raw and jangled, soothing is the key. No sudden movements. No stressful striving.

Of course, for most of us, this is impossible to do all the time. You probably still have to work or take care of family or both, plus whatever else your life involves. It's okay--there's still hope for your recovery.

I will note that for some of us, some of the time, we might need to do a little activity before we can slow down. We might need to yell, shake, or some other action first. When we are at high levels of nervous system activation, it can be challenging to drop to doing nothing all at once. In their book *Burnout: The Secret to Unlocking the Stress Cycle*, Emily and Amelia Nagoski do an excellent job of explaining the physical effects of stress and ways to complete the stress cycle, so I won't duplicate that here.

> *Human Giver Syndrome - the contagious belief that you have a moral obligation to give every drop of your humanity in support of others, no matter the cost to you - thrives in the patriarchy, the way mold thrives in damp basements.*
>
> *- Emily & Amelia Nagoski, Burnout: The Secret to Unlocking the Stress Cycle*

Exercise:

What's one thing you can say no to this week to make a little space for yourself?

Is there some kind of movement, sound, or activity that your nervous system needs before it can start slowing down? Can you let yourself do that thing?

2.5 Scary Scarcity

Many healing professionals start their own practice sometime during their career. Ah, freedom! Setting your own schedule, picking out furniture and fonts, determined that you'll get it right. You'll finally be able to have that work-life balance that you dreamed of while you were struggling as a contractor or employee of someone else.

This is <u>so</u> much harder than it looks. It's hard not to slip into fear. We can get so afraid of scarcity that we contort ourselves to meet every client whim, throwing sustainability out the window.

This happens with schedules in particular. Client can only come in at 8:30 am? Or 8:30 pm? Sure, why not. It's just one day a week, after all. And you need the money. Next thing you know, time after time you're dragging yourself to that appointment, cursing yourself for saying yes.

Or with the types of clients we choose to take on. Maybe you swore you'd never work with teenagers or with diabetes or with divorces, and yet here you are because you feared that nothing else would come along if you turned down this client. Maybe you even find yourself staying silent and downplaying your discomfort when a client acts inappropriately verbally or physically because you're worried about a negative review or losing that money.

First, I want to make sure that you know I can't make any guarantees about your business or your income. None.

What I'm saying is that if you give yourself the gift of being able to build a work life that you want, let yourself have the damm gift! Getting yourself back into a schedule that you hate because you're afraid of scarcity means that not only are you miserable again, you're now dealing with the emotional impact of it being your own doing. Self-betrayal doesn't feel good. It erodes our confidence in our ability to take care of ourselves.

Now imagine that you <u>did</u> let yourself have that work set-up you want. Even if your caseload isn't full, I'm guessing that you'll have more energy to use that open time to do things that will build your business and get you more of your ideal clients in the long run. No one wants to go to a healer who seems miserable and exhausted. Self-care allows you to be more of who you want to be--and who your clients are seeking. I know a helper who usually schedules only one client a day so she can give that client the best possible attention and assistance. Of course, she also had to learn to confidently market her services and charge rates that allow her to keep that schedule, but she has energy to do that because of her small client list. She then gives back to her community by teaching monthly donation-based workshops.

We can also start saying yes to everyone because we're scared of someone saying no to us. Not everyone is going to want to be your client, and that's okay. It doesn't mean that you're not a skilled helper. Some people really like pineapple on their pizza. They can't explain why. They just like it. Just like some people are revolted at the mere mention of pineapple pizza. There's nothing inherently inferior or wrong about either permutation of pizza. It's simply a matter of what we're drawn to. And the people who need your unique style and gifts will be drawn to you.

Because, look—there are piles of books out there on coping with burnout and being a better helper. Something attracted you to this one in particular. As long as you're willing to let yourself be seen and spread the word about your services, your clients will likely be drawn to you, even if it takes a little longer than you were expecting.

We'll talk more about ways to deal with thoughts and emotions like fear in the chapters to follow. You can use those tools with these scarcity thoughts and scared feelings so that you're better able to make decisions from a clear place.

Exercise:

I know you might be pretty drained already. If you can, spend a moment on this exercise.

Visualize your typical start of your work week. Think about how you feel starting your day, your energy level, and anything else about that time.

Now do the same thing with your typical Friday afternoon (or whenever your work week is nearing its end). How do you feel about how you've spent your time this week and the work you've done? Are you ready to run out the door as soon as you can? Are you already dreading the start of the next work week?

Taking it a step further, imagine that the way you feel about your work and the ways you spend your time are going to be the same as they are now for the next 10 years.

What comes up in your body as you consider that? How does your mind react? Do you feel a sense of dread? Of satisfaction?

Is there anything you'd like to change about your work or personal life based on these reflections?

What's one small step you can take towards that change this week?

3. You Can't Fix Them (and why that's a good thing)

3.1 Factors Involved in Change

Helping professions are all about change. The idea is to help people feel better and get them the support and care they need. We can fall into the mindset that we're fixing people—but we can't.

My simple response to why you can't fix them? Because they're not broken. (And neither are you.)

The longer answer has to do with the inherent messiness of being human with a human mind and emotions and ways of interpreting and relating to our experiences. There's so much that you can't change about that, and much that doesn't need to change because it helps us in some way.

If you come at clients like they're a broken chair and you have the hammer, you're not going to get very far, and you might even bash your thumb a few times in the process. If you come at them like you are the only one with all their answers, you're operating on a false assumption and risk disempowering them.

In fact, it's important to deeply accept that you'll NEVER have all the answers. For anyone. Including yourself. Never. *Never ever.* And that's okay. The sooner you let go of that unnecessary and impossible pressure, the sooner you'll be able to be more effective and less frustrated with the people you're helping.

Accepting that no one has all the answers also makes us less likely to become drawn in by someone claiming that they do. Our minds crave simple solutions, clarity, and defined courses of action. Unethical salespeople, abusive teachers, conspiracy theory proponents, cults, and predatory pyramid schemes know this and use it to pull us in with false promises of knowing the answer, the cure.

(By the way, I don't have all the answers either. This book is for you to take or leave as you wish. The only thing I know for sure is how much we can't know.)

The balanced way is for us and our clients to realize that being human is an imperfect business. There's a lot of it we cannot change. We're going to have all kinds of thoughts running through our minds, most of them repetitive and critical. We're going to experience an entire spectrum of emotions, many of them uncomfortable. What we can change is our behavior, if we want to, and with the right help.

And that's where you can come in. You can foster a safe environment that supports exploring change.

There's a good deal of research on how change happens in psychotherapy. You might assume that it's all the fancy therapeutic techniques that have the biggest effect. So you'll be surprised to hear that it's a lot simpler than that.

Psychologists have been researching what makes therapy work for a long time. In that process, they identified certain common factors that seem to make therapy more effective regardless of technique. That's right. No matter what kind of fancy therapy stuff they were doing, these common factors made as much as or more of a difference. These common factors are "therapeutic alliance, empathy, goal consensus and collaboration, positive regard and affirmation, mastery, congruence/genuineness, mentalization and emotional experience" (Nahum et al., 2019).

In other words, the relationship between therapist and client, empathy, agreeing and working together on a common goal, treating your client like you admire and like them, helping them learn how to do things, being real, paying attention to thinking and feeling, and experiencing emotions are the most essential parts of therapy (and other healing work).

The irony here is that when we're caught up in impostor syndrome and feeling like we aren't well-trained enough, it's easy to lose some of these common factors. We have difficulty being fully focused on another person when we're trying to decide what fancy method to use, hoping the client will see us as competent. And if we don't know how to relate to our own emotions, we'll certainly have a hard time sitting with those of others (more on that later).

Reflection:

What comes up for you when you hear the suggestion that you can't fix people and that you won't ever have all the answers?

Which common factors are your strengths? Which could use more of your attention?

3.2 Stages of Change

Thunk. Thunk. Thunk. That sound? It's the sound of healers and helpers feeling like they're hitting a brick wall with clients who can't seem to DO anything. Clients who relapse, who talk about making changes but don't take any actual steps towards change, clients who seem stuck. This frustration and helplessness fuel helper burnout and compassion fatigue.

Near the end of the 1970s, two researchers named Prochaska and DiClemente explored how we humans make changes. After studying smokers' process of quitting smoking, they created the stages of change model, which proposed that the part of change we can see—the actions—are only a tiny part of the change process (Freeman & Dolan, 2001).

Early in the change process, we hang out in the precontemplation stage for a while. We don't have a lot of awareness about the behavior being a problem, and if we think about making a change, it seems like it would be more trouble than it's worth. We're not changing anytime soon, at least not for six months or so. In this stage, we might be okay if someone gave us a little of information on the problem or some referrals to helpers, although we might throw it in a pile and not read it right away. Consciousness raising can be useful here.

Once we become more aware that a problem exists, we might scoot over into contemplation. Now we admit something is going on and that changing soon could be helpful. But we're on the fence about whether we want to put the time and effort into actually making a change. We might talk about it at length with others who could feel frustrated because we're not taking any action. However, this stage is important. Here we need encouragement that we can make the change, that it's possible for us.

 After we've spent some time contemplating the pros and cons, if we decide to make the change, it's time for preparation. Now we plan and lay the internal and external groundwork for change. We might even take small action steps. This stage is a great time to seek professional support.

If we continue on this path, we enter the more visible action stage. We're doing it! Here we go! We are stopping, modifying, or starting some kind of behavior.

Once we do that action stuff for about six months, the initial rush of changing wears off, and it takes maintenance for change to stick. This stage is less glamorous than the action stage. It's the daily work that's needed to prevent relapses and keep the change going in all the situations that we encounter in life. Since maintaining change grows monotonous, this is a stage where support and continuing to celebrate successes can be helpful. (Think of 12-Step programs and the chips that members earn along the way at certain milestones.) Remembering why we made the change in the first place and what life was like before the change can keep us motivated.

Some versions of this model include a termination stage in which we've reached the point where the change is pretty permanent. That's rare. This stage doesn't offer much regarding how to work with clients, so we'll leave it at that.

Here are the things to remember about any kind of stage model. This is a theoretical model that has some research supporting it, but individual results may vary, especially when considering factors such as socioeconomic status.

Also, models are linear. Humans are messy. We jump from stage to stage and back again, sometimes skipping some, sometimes sliding all the way to the starting point. Leave your clients room to be messy and avoid trying to march them through a rigid linear process.

I'm telling you about this model because it helps us broaden our view of the process of change and reduce everyone's frustration. For example, we could spend months butting heads with a client who is in precontemplation because we're using techniques that are better suited for the action stage. Or we can meet them where they are and talk casually about others who have made that change and the pros and cons of it, knowing that we likely won't see action for a while, if ever. And that's okay.

Exploration:

Think of a past or current client who has been frustrating to work with. If you can't bring one to mind, you can use someone from your personal life as an example. What stage of change are they in? What stage have you been approaching them from? Now that you know about the stages of change, what would you change about your work with them?

3.3 Of -isms and Other Issues

*I'm asking if you give advice because you
want to help or if you give advice because
you think you know better. There's a
difference.*

-Nita Brooks, Essence of Perfection

While we're talking about motivation and change, let's reflect on why and how we are drawn to do for others. First, do some self-inquiry into why you're wanting to help. Here are some reasons that might pop up, and if they do, meet yourself with some kindness and then see how you can fulfill that need some other way:

➤ Avoidance of our own problems (sometimes even physically, like working long hours to stay away from home)

➤ Need to feel important

➤ Need to feel needed

➤ Need to feel powerful/capable

➤ Desire to be seen in a certain light

➤ Our own discomfort with someone expressing pain or distress and a desire to make it stop so we feel less anxious or guilty

➤ Excuse for our other less-than-ideal behavior (e.g., I spent 12 hours dealing with crises today, so it makes sense that I canceled on my friend, snapped at my family, spent too much online shopping, and ate an entire cake)

➤ Avoiding feelings of helplessness

➤ Avoiding fears of our own mortality

My energy work teacher Vanessa Stone reminded us that "you can only serve the willing." That phrase helps me when a client isn't receptive to what I suggest. More than that, it's a useful reminder to check in with clients to see what kind of help they are actually seeking before we dive right into interventions. We might assume that someone has certain goals based on our own biases and desires. So use caution and stay in beginner's mind. Their goal might surprise you. For example, some wheelchair users see their wheelchairs as useful tools that bring them freedom and don't consider giving up their chair to be a priority. Some people whose weight is above what charts say it should be are comfortable with their size and may be healthier in terms of fitness than someone who weighs less. Sometimes the problem isn't the condition or disability itself—it's how society responds to it that causes problems (e.g. ableism, lack of accessible accommodations, fatphobia).

Sometimes a client's issue isn't theirs. Something may be broken in their environment, city, country, or culture. If we want to be healers and helpers, we also have to offer help and healing for the problems that go beyond any one individual. All the acupuncture in the world can help support someone's lungs, but if they are breathing smog as soon as they step out the door (or even worse, if they head down into their job in a loosely regulated coal mine the next day), there's only so far that acupuncture can go. A person of color in the current United States is likely never to be totally free of anxiety and stress because living in a country where racism and white supremacy continue to flourish in ways ranging from subtle to blatantly brutal is inherently stressful. You get the picture.

Use particular caution when working with a client who is not the same race as you, especially if you yourself are white. Taking the time to educate yourself on how to be anti-racist can be challenging. However, it is essential if you want to be a truly loving healer. I often wonder if some of the impostor syndrome that so many of us struggle with is fed by the underlying racist system (at least in the United States) that grants unearned advantages and privileges to white people and constantly directly and indirectly tells people of color they are less than.

Another caution arises regarding marketing and selecting your healing practices. There's a tendency among white people in the U.S. (I can't speak to anywhere else) to be drawn to traditional practices of some native peoples, such as shamanism, smudging, plant medicine ceremonies, and so on. Terms like "tribe," "vision quest," and "spirit animal" show up often in certain predominately white circles these days. If you are white, I encourage you to reflect on your activities and the words and images you use to market them. Are you honoring their origins? If you were from that group, how would you feel about someone from another culture using those words or those practices in those ways to make money? Can you take some time to learn about cultural appropriation? What are the traditions and healing practices of your own culture and ancestry (every culture has them) and how can you incorporate or honor those?

Essentially, we can't take ourselves or clients out of the greater context. The more we do our own inner work and work towards social justice, the more healing can happen for all of us.

Reflection:

Take some time to explore the reasons you're driven to help others and what needs that role fulfills for you.

Think about your clients in the larger societal context. What do you need to learn and change in your practice in order to better serve them? What resources can you seek for this? Please do not rely on your client to educate you, since that is asking them for free emotional labor. Continuing education courses, books, videos, and professional consultation are all options for learning.

3.4 Facing Change as a Provider

Arms aching as I struggled up the stairs of my grad school apartment, I finally reached my room. The textbooks bounced on my bed with a plop as they spilled out of my grasp. I picked up the heaviest one, admiring the smooth silver dust jacket. Now I felt like a "real" psychologist.

The *Diagnostic and Statistical Manual of Psychiatric Disorders* is the book that lists all the mental health diagnoses and the criteria for each one. That silver book was the fourth edition, text revised. All of my classes, all of my training, all the seminars that I taught to interns—it was all based on the information and diagnoses in that book. I had it down. Even when I learned about how problematic psychiatric diagnoses are and the issues that underlie deciding what is psychopathology, I still knew the book inside and out.

An indigo book showed up in 2013. The fifth edition of the *DSM*. And so did my resistance. I was shocked at how petulant I felt about it. After all those years learning something else—why did I have to learn a new manual, let alone buy one? I was so stubborn, griping internally when I had to take trainings and finding it harder to learn and remember the diagnostic criteria. Blaming the book, I grew grumpier and grumpier, even complaining about how it went against precedent by switching the edition number from a Roman numeral to an Arabic one. Talk about petty.

What was going on? Was it really such a huge deal? I enjoy learning and have spent decades and tons of money doing it. This was just something else to learn.

On reflection, I think it might have been shame.

Shame that something that had been so easy for me was not coming naturally. Shame that I was having trouble with a basic part of my job at this point in my career.

We have to watch for shame. Early in our careers, we are more likely to expect it. It's later on that it can sneak up on us. If you are unnaturally negative about a change, check for shame. Putting off implementing that change? Check for shame. Avoiding asking for help with that change? You guessed it—check for shame.

No matter what your profession, there is no way that everything about that profession can be known and available at the exact moment of your training. If it was, continuing education wouldn't be a thing. There will always be more to learn, new techniques, new advances, new technology, new equipment. And you'll never ever *ever* be able to learn all of it. And that's okay. If we can come to terms with this reality, it can help shrink that shame. Finding a study buddy colleague who is also struggling with learning something new helps too.

Not knowing something doesn't mean we're a failure as a helper or healer. Not knowing just means that we have the opportunity to continue to become a better and better one.

Exploration:

What's a change in your field that has been challenging for you? How might shame and other emotions be playing a role in that challenge?

3.5 Unsolvable Problems & the Human Condition

Once or twice a year the abbot at the San Francisco Zen Center, Tenshin Reb Anderson, comes to speak with the hospice volunteers. One night he gave a talk that included the best advice I've ever heard on caregiving. He said simply,

"Stay close and do nothing."

That's how we try to practice at Zen Hospice Project. We stay close and do nothing. We sit still and listen to the stories.

- Frank Ostaseski

As helpers and healers, we run up against the frustration of someone not being ready to change behavior, but we can also struggle with internal experiences like thoughts and feelings.

Whether they are our own or someone else's, we can find ourselves exhausted and frustrated.

I propose we drop the struggle.

If a light bulb burns out, you replace it. If the leg falls off your chair, you screw it back on (or decide you want a new chair). If you spill something, you wipe it up. If you put your hand on a hot stove, you take your hand off, quickly. This is how the world works.

Well, that's how the outside world works.

Our inside world is an entirely different place. Down is up and up is sideways. The rules of gravity don't apply here.

In our inside world, the world of thoughts and feelings and some physical sensations, that old saying from the psychologist Carl Jung, "what we resist, persists" is the law of the land. (If you're curious, the full quote is "what you resist not only persists, but will grow in size." He said this in many forms, and the short one is the one that...well, persists.)

You've likely tried not to think about something, perhaps that meeting you have tomorrow or a painful memory. How well did that work? You might have suppressed it for a while, but it came back again, right?

Or have you ever tried not to feel something? Whether it was suppressing the urge to laugh or trying to tune out a wave of grief, I'm guessing you weren't too successful (unless you went numb, which has its own drawbacks).

If getting out of a depressive episode was as easy as "just cheer up," everyone would do that. It's not. And trying might even make the depression a little worse or last longer. Because this is the inside world, and it plays by inside world rules: what we resist, persists.

Both we and our clients can get stuck and frustrated if we use the wrong rulebook. So let's talk about the inside world and how to navigate it.

Drop the struggle. As helpers, we can get caught up in the level of symptoms/feelings/thoughts. At this level, we can fight against them all session long and try to squish them down. Some symptoms can be eliminated, but many, such as chronic pain or deeply ingrained PTSD reactions, might always exist. If we're in the struggle, we're fighting constantly as they pop up over and over, judging our success or failure by whether or not they exist. We all get tired and frustrated.

If we switch to the inside rulebook, we can focus our efforts on how we and our clients cope with and relate to those symptoms/thoughts/feelings rather than spending all our energy trying to eliminate them. That may feel like giving up when you first hear it, but think about it. If you have a client who has been chronically depressed most of their life, what would be more helpful: endlessly trying (and often failing) to reduce their symptoms or helping them get the skills they need to do things that feel meaningful whether or not their symptoms are flaring? And I don't mean in a "suck it up and drive on" kind of way. I mean in a "feel it and thrive" kind of way. What if they could apply those same tools to any emotions or symptoms that they experience in the future?

We can reclaim the energy we used in that struggle and put it towards doing things that make our lives and our work feel more meaningful. What's more, once we start playing by the inside rules, we can stop beating ourselves up for feeling whatever we're feeling. If we can avoid piling shame on top of anger or guilt on top of depression, that saves a lot of heartache.

It can save a lot of heartache for helpers too. We can drop that struggle and take some pressure off of ourselves to stop trying to cure the incurable. But first, we have to learn how, which we'll cover in the next chapters.

Exercise:

Identify a client or situation where you've been stuck in the struggle. What would it be like to drop the struggle? What's been the benefit and the cost of the struggle?

What worries do you have about dropping the struggle?

4. They're Not Broken (and neither are you)

4.1 Humans and Toasters

Let me clarify something.

When I say "they're not broken," I'm talking about emotionally, mentally, spiritually, behaviorally, and so on. Toasters can break and be fixed. However, the essence of a living being isn't broken and we don't need to (and can't) fix it. Humans aren't toasters.

What about bodies, you ask? Bones can break and be set, right? I think bodies fall in a middle ground...there is much that medicine and treatments of various types can do, and then there's always a part of healing that is up to the body itself. A physician can set a bone, but a slew of processes inside the body will determine whether and how and when that bone will knit together. We have little influence over those aspects of healing, especially in other people.

But for the purposes of this book, we'll keep it simple and say "they're not broken."

Now that we've established that, let's turn to a few things for you and your clients to keep in mind when in the process of making any change.

4.2 The Importance of Mercy in Growth

You've accomplished so much already, plus you've gotten this far in the book. You're doing an outstanding job!

What's that? After reading that line, your mind is already prepping a PowerPoint presentation of all the blunders and times you put your foot in your mouth and missed an opportunity, etc., etc., etc.?

And how did I know that? Because that's what minds like to do. They're really worried about our survival, so they are in constant worst-case scenario/training-for-the-end-of-the-world mode. To a survival-focused mind, things like fun and pleasure aren't important, so they're easily glossed over or sometimes even fall right out of our minds.

This mental bias creates problems in other ways. Here are three of them that can grind down our self-compassion.

Myth One: If I'm struggling, it must be because there's something wrong with me or because I'm a bad person.

This one packs such a punch! We're already in pain, then our mind tells us that it's all our own damm fault that we're in pain in the first place. Now we all make mistakes, and sometimes those mistakes lead to painful consequences, but that's different. This is more about when we believe that our pain says something about who we are as people.

We can blame the just-world hypothesis for this one. It has infiltrated American culture (and likely some others). The just-world hypothesis states good things happen to good people, and bad things happen to bad people. Nice and tidy. And a myth. This belief is a mental effort to pretend that the world is predictable and to give us a false sense of control. It's scary to think that sometimes bad stuff just happens and there's nothing we can do about it...at the same time, acknowledging that reality frees us from self-blame and shame.

(As a side note, the just-world hypothesis also drives a lot of victim-blaming and that unsolicited advice we might get from other people or be tempted to give.)

Myth Two: Once I have a full caseload/lose weight/make more money/graduate/find a partner/etc., I'll love myself.

Well, wouldn't that be lovely, if that was all it took? Sorry to smash your dreams, but this isn't how self-compassion and befriending ourselves works. If we "better ourselves" from a place of disdain and self-loathing, even if we accomplish whatever goal we set, we'll still be full of disdain and self-loathing, just maybe in a different cubicle or different clothes.

Contrary to many romantic comedies (and that sneaky just-world hypothesis again!), we don't have to earn love. From anyone. Including ourselves. We are already worthy of love just being born on this planet. See if you can shift to making your self-compassion unconditional. I know you have compassion in you...for baby animals, for your friends, for your clients, for the planet. You have the capacity, you just need better aim.

Myth Three: Everyone else has their shit together, so there must be something wrong with me because I don't.

I have spent about 20 years as a helper in various forms listening to clients' deepest, darkest secrets and shame. I can promise you that NO ONE has their shit together. No matter how polished they may look on the outside, no matter how successful in their craft or work, no matter how popular. Everyone carries their own pain. Their own worries. Their own inadequacies and fears of being an impostor. Their own less-than-helpful behaviors. Everyone.

We just don't talk about it. That's changing a little these days, but it's still more common to hide problems or to hand-pick a few minor ones to polish into "authentic" and "vulnerable" Instagram posts. Especially when you're a helper.

I promise you, anyone who looks like they have their shit together is either dropping some balls in a less visible part of their lives or has someone else juggling some things for them. No one can do it all perfectly, not in this complex day and age.

As a group, healers and helpers often hide our struggles and lack of capacity, so it can feel like you're the only one having a hard time. I assure you, you aren't.

It's hard to shift away from these myths sometimes. I appreciate you giving me a few minutes of open-minded curiosity.

Exploration:

Watch how these myths show up in your own life. Watch how they play out in media and conversations. The first step to any change is awareness.

4.3 Talk to Yourself

We hear it over and over again: "talk to yourself like you'd talk to your best friend." Easy to make into a pretty Instagram post, but hard to do. It is even harder if some of that internal criticism includes echoes from past abusive situations or developed after a traumatic experience. If you're getting overwhelmed trying to figure out where to start to change your self-talk, here are three quick and simple (not necessarily easy) options.

Trick One: Trade Shoulds for Wishes

Just my opinion, but I have almost never found the word "should" to be useful. It makes us feel bad about ourselves or bad about someone else. The word "should" brings on guilt, blame, shame....all kinds of exhausting emotions. Instead, try out using "wish" in its place and see how that works for you. For example, instead of "I should have prepared more for that presentation," try telling yourself, "I wish I had prepared more for that presentation." Instead of "They should have known that I don't like raspberries," try "I wish they had known that I don't like raspberries." It's a little shift, but it's a shift.

Since it's a little shift, this is a simple assignment to give clients early in your work together. We can learn a lot from looking at what we "should" about.

Trick Two: Eliminate Extremes

If you observe it carefully (and if your mind is anything like mine), you'll notice that your self-talk contains a lot of extreme language. Extreme language includes words like "always" and "never." Words like this often signal a false statement--it's almost impossible to always do something or never do something. When you notice an extreme word, experiment with replacing it with something more moderate, like "sometimes," "often," or "tend to." It's a tiny movement that might make a big difference over time.

Trick Three: Replace Apologies with Gratitude

This trick can be used internally with our own self-talk as well as with others around us. It's so easy to fall into apologizing for everything, even things that aren't our fault. Instead of making others feel better, it waters down the power of an apology when it's truly appropriate. Not to mention making us feel smaller and more guilty, and thus more stuck. So, instead of apologizing to the next wall you run into or for needing to use the restroom, try thanking people instead. What would this look like? Say you're running late to a meeting. Instead of the usual "I'm so so so sorry I'm late," try "Thank you so much for your patience" or "I really appreciate your patience."

Using this trick adds the benefit of modeling a more empowered stance for clients. When you tell them, "Thank you for your patience" instead of groveling for being late, you can show them you care about both them and your self worth.

Alrighty, there you have it. Three tricks to shift your language to shift how to talk to yourself and others in order to shift how you feel about yourself.

Exercise:

Try the tricks, either one at a time or all at once, and see how it goes. These kinds of tricks take some time to show their full effect, so don't get discouraged if you don't see a result right away. You're worth investing the time and effort.

5. Noticing

5.1 Mindfulness for Healers and Helpers

You may have heard the word "mindfulness" so many times that you're sick of it, or it might be new to you. Either way, let's look at the role of mindfulness in healing and helping.

Mindfulness is tricky for us helpers. We often tell our clients to practice mindfulness, we teach them mindfulness, and we can give them all kinds of wonderful resources. And then we don't do it. Maybe it's a lack of time. Maybe there's some fear about what we might find if we stay still. We could even feel like we don't need it because we've done it so much over the years, as if we could bank meditation credits for later. Or it might seem like we have been practicing because we talked about it all day with our clients. Whatever the reasons, I suggest you strongly consider revitalizing or beginning your own mindfulness practice. Any kind of mindfulness practice, whether physical or sitting practice, can help us build the muscle to do the work we want to do in a sustainable way.

We can't use our tools efficiently if we don't know what we are using them for. Mindfulness gives us a millisecond to recognize when something is coming up for us, which helps us decide which coping tools to use. It gives us a moment to figure out what's our stuff and our own reactions to a client and what's their stuff. The more aware we are of what's going on inside us while we are working with someone, the more likely we are to be effective and to minimize how much our own biases affect our work.

Mindfulness helps us build our ability to choose our response from a wiser place, not a reactive place. We can better recognize what's going on, and better choose our response.

Mindfulness can also be our little mini break. Like a palate cleanser between clients or at the beginning and end of the day. It's so easy to forget that being in the moment can be a relief sometimes. Not always, of course. But often.

The more that we practice mindfulness, the better we become at modeling this skill for the people we serve. We learn the tricky bits and the ins and outs of this practice, making us better teachers. Having our own practice also can reduce any sense of hypocrisy or impostor syndrome, since we are practicing what we preach.

Exercise:

Try doing a mindfulness practice at least two times this week. There are many guided mindfulness exercises available for free online, and even more on apps. I have several of my own available on the *Insight Timer* app.

Not much time? Here are some ideas for quickie practices (these also appear in *I Can't Fix You*):

Forget How to Do Something: Pretend that you've forgotten how to do something that you do every day, like brush your teeth or make your breakfast. When you do that task, do it with as much attention as you would if you were doing it for the first time. What muscles do you use? What smells or sounds do you notice? Whenever your mind wanders, bring yourself back to the task at hand and your senses.

Three Slow-Motion Bites: This is best done at the beginning or end of a meal, although you can throw them in at any point. Slow down as you approach your food. Look at it, noticing colors, textures, how it catches the light. Smell it. Check in with your body and how it is responding to looking at the food. The mind will probably chime in too, and you can just notice those thoughts as part of the experience. As you take your first bite, pay close attention to the temperature, texture, and flavors that start to emerge. Chew slowly, following the flavors as they shift and change. Wait a second or two longer than you usually would before swallowing, then pay attention to the food as it travels down to your stomach. Give yourself a moment to notice the flavors left in your mouth, then slowly repeat the process with the next two bites.

What's New? This one is great on a busy day. Each time you go into or out of a place that you visit often (this can also include rooms in your house), look for something that you've never noticed before. It can be anything.

CHAPTER SIX

6. Doing the Unstuck

He was alone with his thoughts. They were
extremely unpleasant thoughts and he
would rather have had a chaperon.

-Douglas Adams, Life, the Universe and
Everything

6.1 Why Squishing Doesn't Work

You've probably already tried some things to deal with unpleasant and uncomfortable thoughts. My guess is that you've
thrown affirmations at them, tried to squish them out of exist-
ence, or got to the point where you believed them as fact (and
maybe all of the above).

There's a super-sneaky secret about thoughts: The more we
try to suppress them, the stronger they come back later! Yep,
engaging with our thoughts and trying to argue with them can
actually get us more tangled up in them (Abramowitz et al.,
2001).

Since suppressing thoughts makes them stronger, "the power of positive thinking" can be problematic. Hear me out. Encouraging ourselves, being a cheerleader, imagining good outcomes--all of that is lovely and can be helpful. What I'm talking about here is the belief that's popular in some circles that the wording of our thoughts directly creates our reality. Sure, that sounds great when our mind is giving out shiny happy thoughts, but it can also result in us engaging in constant, exhausting scanning of our brain's secretions, which are naturally going to lean more towards anxious and worried than shiny happy. Evolutionarily, our mind has a negative bias to look for threats in order to keep us safe. Recent research suggests that we have at least 6,200 thoughts a day (Tseng & Poppenk, 2020). That's an awful lot of thoughts to monitor, change, and squish while trying to do everything else that life asks of us.

So what to do?

Reflection:

What have you tried to deal with unpleasant thoughts? What have your clients tried? How well have those strategies worked? What was the cost of using them?

6.2 Cognitive Defusion

This strategy has a fancy name: cognitive defusion. Cognitive defusion means that, with effort and some mindfulness practice, we can get to the point where we can notice and acknowledge a thought without it becoming anything more than a thought. It doesn't seem like reality. We can see that it isn't necessarily a fact. We know that a thought is composed of a bunch of sounds that happen to be considered words in the language that we speak, and we know that these sounds only have as much power and meaning as we choose to give them.

This is damm hard sometimes! Some thoughts are so sticky that we can choose our behavior based on them before we even realize it. They're not actually driving, but we start treating them like the GPS.

But here's another secret: Sure, we can have the GPS on and it can be talking to us. Still, we get to decide whether we follow those directions! We even get to decide whether we listen to it at all. Yeah, it can be distracting and annoying to have it droning on in the background, but we're still driving where we have chosen to go, making changes and choices all along the way.

Here's an example. If you've ever driven on the highway I-35 in Texas, you know well the mysterious traffic jams that come out of nowhere and last for hours. Sometimes there's an actual event like an accident that blocks the lane, but sometimes these slowdowns have no apparent cause and it seems like there's just a glitch in the space-time continuum. This time I hit one of these around Waco the night before Thanksgiving. I had Google Maps giving me directions, but then I turned on the Waze app to get a better prediction of the traffic situation. My Waze app had the Cookie Monster voice; my Google Maps app was set on a feminine voice with a British accent. I was slowly weaving my way through Waco side streets when they started telling me to do different things. One was saying go one way, the other was telling me the opposite, and Cookie Monster was throwing in some intense demands for me to stop and buy cookies. (I shit you not. My GPS was telling me to buy cookies.)

So what did I do? I spotted a familiar landmark and chose to go a completely different way. Both apps erupted into blips and commands to do this and turn there and try to get back on their routes, but I kept going on the route that I had chosen. Eventually the voices settled down and caught onto my plan-- although it was really noisy for a hot minute. (And no, I did not buy cookies. Cookies are delicious, but there was no time to stop and shop.)

This is what happens in our head when we try to do something new, or do anything that has some risk in it, whether it's start a private practice or call that potential client back. Our internal GPS freaks out and tells us to turn around, getting louder and louder until we either do what it says—or we keep going on our own path for long enough that it gives up and gets with the program.

How to ride it out?

Play a little

Using metaphors like seeing those thoughts as a GPS or as coming from a cartoon character can help us laugh at them and take them less seriously. Humor is a powerful unsticking agent. You can also try saying them out loud in a funny voice or singing them like you're in a musical or opera.

Say thanks

You might think of these thoughts (whew, that's a bit meta) as misguided but well-meaning folx. You can politely thank them without acting on any of their "advice." I personally use "Thanks for sharing!" as my response to unhelpful thoughts.

Remember that they're just thoughts

Putting the phrase *I'm noticing I'm having the thought that...* in front of sticky thoughts gives us a sliver of space so we can choose our behavior rather than automatically following the thought.

The boot on the cover of this book comes from an experience I had in graduate school. Sitting in psychopathology class, of all places, I kept getting a vivid thought that I needed to take off my boot and throw it through the classroom window. Week after week, my mind told me that I had to do this act that would 1) ruin my favorite pair of boots, 2) bring my professional future into question, and 3) put me even further in debt for damages to a state government building. You can imagine I started self-diagnosing and freaking out. That is, until I realized that even after all these weeks of my mind's Throw the Boot campaign, I had never thrown the boot. I didn't have to do everything my mind said, no matter how persistent and vivid the thoughts might be.

And neither do you. You don't have to throw the boot.

Put it on repeat

You know that thing that happens when you write or see a word over and over and you start questioning whether it really is a word? Repetition dissolves language to its barest essence: sounds. After all, language is just a bunch of sounds that everyone who speaks that language has agreed mean a particular thing. We built language, and we can take it apart again. Even the words that feel poky or painful. I'm not saying that words aren't powerful or that we shouldn't pay attention to what we say. I'm just suggesting that if your mind is using certain words that have you feeling awful about yourself, repetition can reduce their power.

Name those reruns

Our minds aren't super-original. They repeat words, and they also repeat entire stories about us. Say there's a story that your mind tells every time you see an email from your supervisor. The story goes something like "I screwed up, I'm getting fired, I'll never be good enough, I'm a horrible failure..." We could give this one the title "The Tale of Terrible Failure." Or "Doom Time." Call it anything you want. Then when you notice those stories popping up, it's easier to name them and work on getting unstuck instead of following them closely.

You can find more about these cognitive defusion techniques in *I Can't Fix You*, along with some examples. Now let's look at how to use defusion with impostor syndrome.

Experiment:

What's one of your common sticky thoughts? Select two of these cognitive defusion strategies and try using them with that thought. What do you notice? Keep in mind that different strategies work better than others for some people and with some thoughts, and the strategies tend to be more effective with repetition.

6.3 Example: Defusing Impostor Syndrome

Almost everyone I know deals with some form of impostor syndrome: the thought that we're not good enough for that job, that we don't deserve that award, that we don't know what we're talking about. These thoughts can get pretty darn loud and shouty sometimes, such as when we get close to a goal or have a big accomplishment. If you think about it, you can probably predict the kinds of situations that will trigger your own impostor syndrome thoughts.

We can escape falling into that pit by using cognitive defusion techniques. Like anything, different ones work for different people at different times. Here are a few ways you could do this with the thought I'm a fraud.

Play a little: Sing *I'm a fraud* over and over to the tune of a song, like *Twinkle Twinkle Little Star*, or make up your own tune. (I'm partial to singing thoughts Broadway-style myself.) Alternatively, you could say it in the lowest or highest voice you can comfortably manage every time it goes through your mind.

Say thanks: If we take the stance that our mind cares about us but is worried and overprotective, we can look at impostor syndrome thoughts as ineffective ways that our mind is trying to save us from failure or embarrassment. And then we can express our gratitude for the concern—while ignoring its advice. "Thanks, mind! I know this is a bit of a risk, but I think we're prepared to handle whatever happens." Or you could simply say, "Thanks for sharing! I appreciate the input."

Remember that they're just thoughts. Here's where we can throw that phrase *I'm noticing I'm having the thought that* in front of *I'm a fraud*. Doing so takes us from *I'm a fraud* to *I'm noticing I'm having the thought that I'm a fraud*. Try both on and see how each of them feels.

Put it on repeat. For this one, you can speak it or write it. Either way, the key is to repeat the phrase over and over as fast as you can for about a minute. You can shorten the time if the thought becomes less sticky before a minute is up. Ready? Here you go: *I'm a fraud, I'm a fraud, I'm a fraud, I'm a fraud, I'mafraudI'mafraudI'madraud...*

Name those reruns: These kinds of thoughts often travel in packs. Perhaps your mind says something like: *I'm a fraud, I have no idea what I'm doing, who am I to be seeing this client/teaching this/leading this workshop, I can't possibly ask people to pay me for my services, I don't deserve to be here.* It's so easy to get caught up in all the individual thoughts. If we group them together, then we have only one to step back from. Giving this cluster of thoughts a name like "The Impostor Story" or "The One Where I'm Fooling Everyone and They're Going to Find Out" can give us just a little more space from the thoughts, improving our chances of getting unstuck. We can say to ourselves, "Oh look! 'The Impostor Story' is on again," and try to let it play out in the background while we swing our attention to something else.

All of this takes practice to become a habit. Our natural tendency is to want to fight the thoughts, to argue with them. Keep reminding yourself that you want to politely acknowledge them, then turn your attention elsewhere. Almost like at a social gathering where you pleasantly nod at someone but stay in your current conversation...or maybe it's more like you are trying to talk on the phone while a five-year-old child is pulling at you to watch them do their latest trick, look at the picture they drew, and tie their shoes. Cognitive defusion uses the same muscles that noticing and mindfulness do. They all invite us to pick a focal point and then bring our attention back to it over and over again, no matter how many times we are distracted. The more we practice this, the stronger that muscle becomes and the better we can aim our attention where we want it, moving it back each time it gets pulled away.

7. Becoming Spacious

*Through it all, the mountain just sits,
experiencing change in each moment,
constantly changing, yet always just being
itself.*

*It remains still as the seasons flow into
one another and as the weather changes
moment by moment and day by day,
calmness abiding all change.*

-Jon Kabat-Zinn

7.1 Zoom: Self-as-Context

There's room for all of it.

Seriously. There is. Everything that you've ever experienced in your life, everything that you ever will experience, everything that you've heard and felt, every client story, all of it.

There's room for all of it for two reasons. First, as I'll talk about more in the next chapter, much of it can flow through and out. Second, we are spacious, endlessly spacious.

You may have heard metaphors about this, such as you're the sky and everything else is just clouds. Or you're the ocean and your feelings are the waves. It's that idea. The idea that your core, true self is indestructible and sits at the center while experiences, thoughts, emotions, sensations, while all of that swirls around it. We can feel it all, but it can't destroy us.

Acceptance and Commitment Therapy (ACT) uses the metaphor of a chessboard. Chess is a two-player game played on a board covered in black and white squares. The players have black or white pieces that they move in certain ways to try to get all the other player's pieces off of the board. For the purposes of this metaphor, the board is infinite, going on and on in every direction.

Chess is a battle between the pieces. In each encounter, one of them is going to "die" (get removed from the board). For the pieces, this is life or death.

When we get caught up in thoughts, emotions, sensations, experiences, or memories, and we try to fight them off or suppress them, we are living at the level of the pieces. We are living in that life-or-death intensity and exhaustion. It's the same thing if we are at that level with our clients, trying to change or counter every single painful thought or emotion they have.

But what if we shift our focus? What if we remember our and their spaciousness and realize that we are actually that infinite, indestructible board? The board has plenty of room for all of it. The board feels the battles going on, but it doesn't have to do anything about them. It's an observer, watching it all and taking what is useful from it. And through it all, it remains intact.

The board never runs out of room. Have you ever thought to yourself, "I can't take one more thing"? Well, if you're the board, you can. Sure, you might need some self-care time or some rest to attend to your physical body, but you can take one more thing. Look at everything in your life that you've survived, at all the pieces on your board. You have always found room for it, even if it was excruciating to experience at the time. You've made it through all of it.

If you can get a sense of this spaciousness for yourself, your clients can tell. They'll feel more comfortable with you, even if they can't say why. You'll also feel more comfortable with them, knowing that nothing can emotionally destroy you, that you have room for all that you experience. And hey, you might even get to teach them that their core self is indestructible and infinite too.

(If you like, you can refer clients to Chapter 5 of *I Can't Fix You*, which describes this as the *Zoom* key.)

Exercise:

Practice noticing when you or your clients are operating at the piece level and see what it's like to expand your focus and sense of self to the infinite board level. See if that can give you a little breathing room. A consistent mindfulness meditation practice can help enhance this skill.

7.2 Co-regulation

*When you begin to touch your heart or let
your heart be touched, you begin to
discover that it's bottomless, that it doesn't
have any resolution, that this heart is
huge, vast and limitless. You begin to
discover how much warmth and gentleness
are there, as well as how much space.*

-Pema Chödrön

This *Zoom* key, remembering that you have space for all of it, is a vital part of co-regulation. You've probably experienced co-regulation at some point in your life. Maybe you went to someone for support when you were really upset and agitated, possibly even yelling.

Now imagine that they started yelling and acting agitated too. You might feel validated at first, like they understood your feelings. But over time, you might notice that you're still just as upset, if not more, than you were when you first went to them.

Let's look at a different version of this scenario. You're still upset, you still went to someone for support, but this time they don't start yelling and getting upset too. They listen attentively and with curiosity, say things that make you feel like they understand your feelings, and they keep a calmer body posture and tone.

In this situation, you might gradually start lowering your volume, breathing more slowly, or becoming more still. Other, quieter feelings might come up, like hurt or sadness, or even a lightening of your mood.

This is co-regulation. We all affect each other. This gives healers the opportunity to help someone make a shift simply by being present in an intentional way. Please remember that I'm not talking about invalidating someone's feelings or ignoring their distress by telling them to calm down! Validation and attention are vitally important to this process. We meet people where they are, but in such a way that we are a model for where they might like to be.

Working with trauma survivors, I have sometimes heard my newer clients express concern and reluctance to tell me about something horrible they experienced for fear that they'll harm me in some way or that I won't be able to handle it. The better we get at becoming spacious, the more confidently we can tell these clients that they can tell us anything--and the more likely they are to believe it.

When you're with a client and feeling a little overwhelmed by their pain or story, try the *Zoom* skill. You might even try opening up your posture: making space between the shoulders and the ears, keeping the palms open, looking for some spaciousness in the chest. Remember how spacious your infinite self truly is! Your experience in that moment with that client is one tiny piece on your chessboard, and no matter how much noise it makes or how much it stomps around, it cannot even scratch the board. Being able to *Zoom* will give you the space you need to co-regulate with intention.

8. It's Not Yours to Hold

8.1 What Goes in Must Come Out

There's another way to think about becoming spacious. Nothing in nature goes in without something coming out eventually. We are not made to hold things forever. And we're not meant to be a holding tank for clients' emotions and trauma! That's not even helpful for them. It's not modeling ways of being with emotions without being overwhelmed. Besides, if we keep holding their stuff long enough, we'll start to consciously or unconsciously want to avoid that client and be less present. It's not ours to hold.

There's an episode (Season 5, Episode 9) of the TV show *30 Rock* in which the earnestly helpful NBC page Kenneth listens to Liz's deep, dark secrets. After spilling her shame and pain, she bounces away, relieved, leaving Kenneth reeling and turning to Jack to share his own trauma, who turns to Tracy Jordan, creating a "chain reaction of mental anguish." Everyone is feeling lighter after talking about their pain, but to keep feeling good, they start dodging people, worried that if anyone talks to them, that person's problems will burst the bright bubble.

And that's what happens to us if we keep taking things in without realizing that we are a pipe, a channel. We get full. We get full, and we get wary of connections for fear that they will add something else to our pile.

Exploration:

Can you relate to this example from *30 Rock*? In what situations do you do this most?

8.2 Let it Flow

*You have a choice whether to open or
close, whether to hold on or let go,*

*whether to harden or soften, whether to
hold your seat or strike out.*

*That choice is presented to you again and
again and again.*

-Pema Chödrön

So we need to find ways to let it flow through us. As it moves through, we can notice our reactions and glean whatever information we need from it, then let it continue on its way. Think of it like the digestive system, where the body extracts the necessary nutrients, then ditches the rest. We're just a conduit.

Where can it go? Well, the earth can handle it. It has tons of room. It might sound cheesy, but you could visualize the energy and emotions as liquid moving down from your ears and eyes and heart through your torso, down your body, and out whatever part of you is closest to the ground. With each exhale, let more of it move through and out. Through and out. You can even do this while the other person is still with you--it's an invisible process. And once you get into the habit of it, it takes very little attention to keep the flow going.

Like with any pipe, there are certain things that are harder to move through than others. These might be:

➢ Painful experiences that you've never considered or heard of before

➢ Experiences or emotions that bump up against your own tender places

➢ Intense material on a day when you're already feeling raw and depleted

➢ Intense material from multiple clients in a row with no breaks

➢ Material related to situations that bring up your own sense of helplessness, such as problems with agencies or systems that you can't easily change

➢ Emotions projected onto you or regarding something about you

➢ Situations that bring up feelings of impostor syndrome

Knowing your own sensitive spots can help you get a little better at predicting potentially tough sessions so you can plan some coping ahead of time. Once you know them, it's time to figure out which tools work best for you. Some options:

➢ **Movement** (yoga, dancing, weightlifting, gardening, sports, running, shaking, rolling around on the floor, swimming, etc.)

➢ **Sound** (singing, screaming, humming, babbling nonsense syllables, chanting, talking to others, playing an instrument, etc.)

➢ **Making** (cooking/baking, crafts, writing, building, fixing things, programming/coding, inventing, etc.)

➢ **Stillness** (restorative yoga, meditation, baths, TV, movies, reading, sleep, massage, etc.)

➢ **Connection** (hugs, talking with a friend, doing a kindness for someone, playing games together, talking to a therapist, etc.)

Exercise:

What are two of your tender spots?

What are three tools you can use to cope?

8.3 Tips for Self-Soothing

There's no magic way to feel awesome during a tough moment, so I'd like to offer what tips I can that might help at least a little here and there.

Remember: the effectiveness of these tips will vary, and none of them will make a feeling or anxiety go away for good. However, practicing them regularly over time may help prevent stress and anxiety from building up to overwhelming levels. And if one of these gets you through 30 seconds, that's 30 seconds more relief than you had before!

The theory here is if we do the things that our bodies naturally do when we're at ease, it can send feedback to the body that we're relatively safe. I've sorted it into Head, Shoulders, Knees & Toes to make it a little easier to remember. (And now you just might have that song in your head. You're welcome.)

Note: I mention several body parts here. If a tip involves one that your body doesn't have access to, modifications include either visualizing yourself doing the action or using a different body part to do that action.

HEAD:

Eyebrows (and the other facial muscles): **Take a few** seconds to move the facial muscles by wagging the eyebrows, making silly faces, scrunching up your face, etc.

Eyes: Let your gaze slowly and casually wander around your surroundings. The movement of the eyes is key here, not the head. This can be combined with some mindful noticing of textures, colors, light, and other visual details.

Nose: Extending the exhale to twice as long as the inhale, keeping the breath very smooth and slow.

Mouth: A closed-mouth tiny smile (like the Mona Lisa) can create a physical shift over time.

Chin: Bringing the chin lower than the forehead is a signal to relax.

Throat: Chewing calms the body, signaling the body to rest and digest. You can chew on food, gum, hard candy, or non-food items like sensory chewies (search online for terms like "sensory chewies" or "chewy fidgets").

Voice: Inhale through nose, then exhale while making the sound *Voo* low and long until you run out of breath. Find a tone and note that feels like an internal massage. Repeat a few times. I've included a link to a demonstration video in the Resources section at the end of the book.

SHOULDERS:

Shoulders: Can you create more space between your shoulders and your ears? Roll the shoulders a few times if that feels good, or bring them up towards the ears, squeeze tightly, then release.

Arms (and other limbs): Make big gestures, keep hands open instead of in fists.

Arms: Do a Butterfly Hug by crossing arms and alternating tapping your chest or upper arms with your hands. (link to video in Resources section). You can go faster than the video does if that feels good to you in that moment.

KNEES:

Knees (and legs): Is there a motion that your body wants to make? Does it want to move quickly or even run away? Does it want to dance, roll, stretch, throw, grab, push, pull, skip, etc.? Can you find a safe and non-harmful way to let it have what it wants for a few minutes? If the motion it wants isn't possible for your body, can you take a little time to vividly imagine doing that motion?

Legs: Getting our legs up above our heart can feel calming and restorative. This doesn't have to involve a handstand! Just putting our calves on the seat of a chair or couch is plenty to get the effect. Learn more here.

TOES:

Feet and toes: Especially if you're feeling frozen, slow and gentle movements can be key. Gradually start wiggling the toes, starting very slowly. Over a few minutes you can move into moving the feet and ankles, staying gentle and smooth.

Other Tricks:

Chill out (literally): Putting an ice pack or cold cloth over the eyes can help calm down the nervous system. Holding an ice cube for a little while (but not so long that you hurt yourself!) can shock you out of an overwhelmed state. If it's okay with your doctor, a cold shower can have a similar effect.

Loving-Kindness Meditation: This meditation can help with self-compassion but is also excellent to use before going into a social situation. There are many free guided versions out there on apps like Insight Timer and on YouTube.

iRest Yoga Nidra: This type of guided meditation is used to help teach the body to relax deeply. There are lots of guided versions available (see Resources section). Some even include a progressive muscle relaxation to create an even greater effect. This meditation can be useful when going to sleep, during a nap, or when you wake up too early and can't fall back asleep. At first, you may find it very difficult to be still and to follow along. That's to be expected if you've been running at full tilt for a long time. Remember that this is a process of teaching the body how to slow down. It won't happen immediately. You're building a relaxation muscle.

Exercise:

Pick three of the tips in this section and try them this week.

8.4 Managing Triggers at Work

Many of us helpers are carrying around our own wounds. Just like our clients, we can encounter situations that trigger old physical or emotional pain. Facing triggers at work can feel extra-challenging due to worries about maintaining a professional reputation, keeping your job, and looking competent. If you don't have a supportive coworker who knows that you're dealing with PTSD, being triggered at work can also feel lonely and isolating. You're not the only one dealing with this and here are some strategies that have helped others like you cope.

Grounding

There are many ways to ground ourselves after being startled or triggered. Grounding reminds us where and when and who we are. Our senses can help with this. Start naming to yourself things around you that you can see/hear/touch/smell. You might even keep a few items handy to help with this, like strong mints, an essential oil or cologne to smell, a fidget cube or small stone to touch, or bookmark some cute videos to watch.

Sometimes reminding ourselves of the date can help, since the traumatic event occurred in the past. Maybe you have a piece of technology, jewelry, or even a hair color or tattoo that didn't exist at the time of the trauma. That can help remind you you're in the present now, not back in the event.

Go Soft and Slow

Being triggered can feel like being inside a shaken snow globe, with bits of artificial snow flying all around you. The glittery fake snow bits will settle back down with time. You can aid in this process by approaching the next few minutes/hours/days gently, as if you are recovering from the flu or a bad sprain. Your nervous system is already on high alert. Remind it that you're in a safer situation now through things like moving slowly and smoothly, allowing yourself to rest when you can, and smoothing out your breathing. As you inhale through the nose, imagine you're smelling something wonderful, and as you exhale gently through the mouth, imagine you're blowing on a spoonful of soup and trying not to spill it. Longer exhales are calming for the body.

If you have a chance to make the space around you softer, do that too. Turn down the volume and brightness on screens or find some sounds that are soothing to you (I like exploring the dozens of sounds on www.mynoise.net).

Make Space

Along the same lines, make yourself some space however you can. If you're lucky enough to be able to take a little time off of work or adjust your schedule, that's wonderful. If you can't, see if you can ask someone to take over a task or to cover while you take five or ten minutes in the bathroom, out back, in your car, in an empty room—anywhere you can take a little space.

If you can't get space at work, maybe you can after work. Can a plan be canceled? Can you ask a friend or family member to help with a task so you can rest for a bit?

If you can't find space that way either, maybe you can plan some for your next day off, or escape into listening or watching something with headphones on so you can feel like you're in your own bubble for a bit, even if you still have to cook or do other chores. If you go the headphones route, make sure the people around you know to avoid coming up to you suddenly so you don't get startled. Being triggered can be exhausting, and it's really common to want a little time alone afterward.

I hope you can hear the common themes through these suggestions: you're not the only one, it's not unusual to feel upset after being triggered, and treat yourself as gently and kindly as you can during the recovery time. We can't avoid triggers completely, but we can get better at taking care of ourselves after being triggered. Then, like with so much of what we learn in life, we can teach it to our clients.

Exercise:

If being triggered is common for you, create a coping plan ahead of time. Where and when can you find space? What or who will you need while you're recovering?

9. You're Indestructible

9.1 The Purpose of Emotions

*Negative emotions like loneliness, envy,
and guilt have an important role to play in
a happy life; they're big, flashing signs
that something needs to change.*

-Gretchen Rubin

*We cannot selectively numb emotions,
when we numb the painful emotions, we
also numb the positive emotions.*

-Brené Brown

I know, you came into healing and helping because you could see how much pain and suffering exist in the world. And you wanted to help ease it, maybe even eradicate it. It feels so darn good when we can help someone feel better (notice that I did NOT say "make someone feel better." More on that later.). We feel warm and fuzzy; they feel warm and fuzzy. So wonderful.

But not entirely wonderful.

See, pain has a purpose. It's a signal that something needs our attention, whether it's our finger or our love for someone. All emotions are messengers that want to tell us something. If we didn't have them, we'd be missing out on vital information, like the handful of people in the world who have the rare genetic disorder called Urbach-Wieth disease. This disease affects the amygdala area of the brain and impairs their ability to experience fear and to recognize it in others. People who have this disease frequently end up in dangerous situations and being hurt because their body and brain don't send a fear signal to remind them to avoid threats (Fessenden, 2015).

Physical pain is also important to our well-being, as much as we'd like to be rid of it. A tiny number of people suffer from a genetic disorder called congenital insensitivity to pain, or CIP. They literally cannot experience physical pain, resulting in numerous severe physical injuries or even death at a young age. When interviewed, they tend to express distress that they don't feel pain, that they have to constantly guess at what might be dangerous for them (Cox, 2017).

Clearly emotional and physical pain are essential. Perhaps the real problem isn't the pain—it's how we relate to it. And our reaction to our clients' pain affects their relationship with their own pain. If we dismiss it, ignore it, try to eradicate it immediately, or freak out about it, they'll either do the same themselves or they'll never come back to see us.

Now simple pain, like if someone has a splinter in their finger, we can take care of swiftly and effectively. Pull out the splinter, clean off finger, feel relief, done. Nice and neat.

The pain I'm talking about here is emotional pain. Pain from thoughts and feelings. From memories. From chronic illnesses and injuries that have no cure. From grief about things that can never be. That kind of messy, unsolvable pain.

This unsolvable pain is the kind we really need to be able to witness. Your clients and others in your life will thank you for it.

Here's the tricky bit: in order to relate to our clients' pain in a helpful way, we have to be able to sit with our own pain first. If you thought this book was going to help you get out of having to do that, sorry. There's truly no sustainable way around it.

Here's the good news: As you learn tools like the ones in the following chapters, you'll be getting a bonus. You can use these strategies with yourself, with clients, and in both personal and professional settings. Nothing wasted, nothing lost. Just a whole lot of freedom to gain.

Exploration:

How has your pain served you? How has it served your clients?

9.2 Other People's Critters

No feeling is forever. Really. Even a feeling that seems to be hanging around for a long time fluctuates constantly. Depression and anxiety levels increase and decrease throughout a day, throughout each hour.

Feelings can't destroy you. Only the actions you choose to take when you have those feelings can. You and your clients have lived through every single emotion you've ever had in your entire life. We healers can be just as scared and avoidant of emotions as our clients are, perhaps even more so since the helper role is a great place to hide out and distract ourselves from our own inner state by focusing on that of others. (Hey, I only know because I've been there. I'm not shaming anyone for it. We're all just human and doing the best we can at the time.)

I won't lie, sitting in the room with someone's pain can feel overwhelming sometimes. There's a reason that many people do not decide to go into helping professions. It's really hard. We have to learn how to cope with our own messy human experience and then figure out how to deal with someone else's and then figure out how to manage the reactions we have to dealing with someone else's pain. That's a lot of layers.

How to do this? First, we have to *Zoom*. And I'm not talking about video calls. We have to be able to *Zoom* out and get in touch with our biggest self, remembering that we have room for all of it. Once we sense our spaciousness, we can sit with our client's pain without it taking us over.

Getting big and spacious goes against our instincts when we're facing something uncomfortable, so it takes practice. Our instinct is often to contract, to curl up in a ball and defend ourselves against the pain. Unfolding to face it? That's like a firefighter learning to run towards the burning building. We can't put out the pain, but we can be a solid presence while our clients ride those waves.

But what does this whole sitting with emotions thing look like? What do you do while you're sitting?

Here's one option based in ACT that you can use yourself and teach to your clients. I use the acronym **WOE** since it's usually the uncomfortable and sadder emotions that are tough for us. Remember to *Zoom* out before you do this—it helps to have that sense of being indestructible when you go to sit with emotions. Now for the acronym.

W: Where is it? Scan to determine where the emotion or sensation is located in your body.

O: Objectively observe the critter, using all your senses.

E: Expand, willingly welcoming the critter(s), knowing you have room for this feeling and many more.

Where is it?

Your emotions aren't in your head. They are a physical experience, so you have to look in your body to find them. If you're finding something with a lot of words, it's a thought, not an emotion. Emotions are an experience. For example, "I feel like you don't care about me when you forget to start the dishwasher" is a thought. Lonely, frustrated, and anxious are emotions.

Emotions can show up anywhere in the body, and everyone experiences them differently. Some common places for emotions to hang out? Check the jaw, shoulders, throat, chest, gut, hands, and legs, particularly the knees.

Objectively observe

Once you've located the critter, imagine that you are gently pulling it out of your chest or wherever it's located to float in the air in front of you. I know that sounds a little kooky, but since emotions don't live in the land of language, we sometimes have to find some creative ways to interact with them. Now that you're watching the critter, observe it as objectively as you can. Describe it to yourself as if you're a scientist who's just discovered this thing.

This is where the senses come into play. What color is it? How big is it? Is it in motion or is it still? What's its temperature? What kind of texture does it have? If it made a sound, what sound would it make? You might even ask yourself what it would taste like. Be as descriptive as you can, going through all the senses.

Note: The mind will want to tell a story about what all this means and worry about why this sensation is present and how long it will stay and what it says about you that you're having it, etc. See if you can let the mind's commentary be background noise and refocus on your senses. Refocus as many times as you need to.

Expand

Once you have observed the first critter, look through your body and see what you notice as you're watching that critter. See if you can locate another emotion or sensation. Once you do, pull that one out and go through the same process. Let it float next to the first critter. And then do it all again with a third one. Now that you have all three critters there where you can watch them, pay attention to whatever feelings or sensations arise while you do that. You can choose in any moment to open your eyes and distract yourself if you need to. Remind yourself that you have experienced many, many big emotions and sensations in the past, and survived them all.

Okay. Here comes the tricky bit. We didn't pull them out to get rid of them (although you might have hoped so). We pulled them out so we could get to know them a little better. And now that we've observed them, now that we've gotten in touch with the fact that we are humans experiencing those emotions and those emotions aren't all that we are, it's time to allow them back in. Well, not even allow them back in, because they have been there all along. I'm not asking you or your client to do anything that you're not already doing. You're already having that emotion, and you're already surviving that emotion.

In expanding, we are allowing ourselves to get big and broad and welcoming. It's like we reach out and scoop those emotions back in, embracing those critters. The key to this is remembering that they can't destroy us. No emotion can destroy us. We have so much room inside.

When working with clients, we can WOE the experience of sitting with them, then WOE the emotions that come from observing their emotions. There are a lot of layers to this, like looking in those sets of mirrors that create infinite reflections. Even when you feel lost in it all, you're still indestructible you at the very core.

This process creates an opportunity to develop a relationship with emotions and sensations. We can even give them personalities and nicknames. It's easier to communicate about and relate to a cold, slow-moving grey blob named Bleh-Bleh than to a nebulous feeling. We can talk to others about Bleh-

Bleh, see if Bleh-Bleh has something to tell us, easily notice that Bleh-Bleh is getting loud and hanging around a lot recently, and then take appropriate coping steps.

Exercises like this give us the ability to sit in the midst of an emotion or sensation and not feel compelled to do anything to make it go away. If we can manage to do this, with practice we learn we don't have to immediately jump to a solution for an emotion. We also become much better able to be present for our clients' emotions and reactions.

If the idea of sitting with emotions still sounds scary to you or your client, think about this. According to Dr. Jill Bolte-Taylor (2008), a Harvard-trained neuroanatomist, unless something re-triggers it, a raw emotion lasts only 90 seconds. Yep. Only 90 seconds. Less than two minutes. That means that if we can keep from interfering with an emotion, refrain from piling suffering on top of pain, it may very well run its course faster and be less distressing in the long run. Techniques like the WOE process can help us get through those 90 seconds without messing with the emotion or adding to it. Of course, if a situation is ongoing, the emotion may return, but we can get through it 90 seconds at a time.

Earlier in this book, we talked about fear of scarcity and how it can drive us to make decisions that aren't healthy for us--if we do what fear says. We don't have to let fear drive, though. The concepts and exercises throughout this book, like this one, can help us make our own decisions and take the wheel back from fear.

Often we or our clients can be tempted to run from emotions, to squish them or to ignore them. We can also be tempted to run from our client's emotions. And that makes us protective, defensive, feeling like we need to avoid people who are in pain for fear that they will somehow drag us down, or steal our energy, or infect us with their darkness. We become like the characters in the *30 Rock* episode described earlier in this book, not wanting to risk an interaction. Think about that slogan "good vibes only." In theory, it seems cheerful and motivating. In practice, what is it telling us and our clients? It's telling us that we are not allowed to be whole here, that we are not allowed to be our full human selves in this place.

But if we are able to zoom out, if we can stay in touch with our indestructible core, and we recognize that no matter how many critters are in the room we can't be destroyed and that they will come and go, then we're able to welcome all vibes. We're able to welcome all that our clients are, all of their experiences. We're able to be better and more sustainable healers and helpers. And isn't that why you're reading this book in the first place? Let's start thinking resilient instead of positive.

Now you might be wondering about this whole emotions can't destroy us thing. If we're sitting in a chair and experiencing an emotion, it will affect us, but it won't destroy us. If we experience that emotion and we decide to jump through the window, then our behavior might destroy us. The choices we make when we experience an emotion can destroy us. But not the emotion itself.

The same goes for our clients. At first, we may have to show them by our example that we can be in the presence of pain and not fall apart. Over time, we can teach them how to do this for themselves, much like we might teach them physical therapy exercises, recipes, or acupressure points to use at home. Being able to sit with emotions without having to scramble to make them go away is a superpower. If we can do that, we can face just about anything.

Over time, you may develop a stance for yourself when you're willing to sit with whatever emotions are coming up within you or someone else. Such a stance involves openness in whatever form that takes in your body—perhaps it is hands, or chest, or arms. Combine that openness with a grounded, sturdy way of sitting or standing, and you have a winning combination ready to WOE.

And yes, it's still okay to dive into distraction sometimes, ideally after you've already taken a few moments to see what the feelings want to tell you. The difference is that we can mindfully choose distraction from an empowered place instead of feeling like we have no other option but to run scared.

Exercise:

Try the WOE technique with a neutral or pleasant emotion for practice. When you feel you have it down, then try it with a slightly uncomfortable emotion (not your most overwhelming one).

Reflection:

In what ways might you have inadvertently conveyed to clients that they're too much? What messages do your marketing and decor send?

10. Are You Willing?

10.1 Humility

*Truly, we live with mysteries too marvel-
ous to be understood...*

*Let me keep my distance, always, from
those who think they have the answers.*

*Let me keep company always with those
who say*

*'Look!' and laugh in astonishment, and
bow their heads.*

-Mary Oliver

As healers, we are asked to simultaneously hold space for the worst potential outcomes and for ever-present hope. We are asked to go headlong into situations that evoke our own grief and loss of innocence as we witness some of the worst things that humans and bodies can do.

To do this work, and certainly to do it well, we must be willing. Willingness is a stance of being open to whatever comes. Willingness isn't just torturing ourselves for no reason;

it is choosing to do so in service of something important to us. When we greet a new client, we are practicing at least a little willingness. Here we are agreeing to meet a stranger in order to help them with problems we won't fully know until we get into the appointment because it is important to us to be helpful.

To listen is to lean in softly

With a willingness to be changed

By what we hear.

-Mark Nepo

Willfulness shows up when we resist the reality of a situation. We might be full of willingness when we work with clients, but then get willful about not asking for help from colleagues or family. Willful looks like railing against the car in front of you for not going the speed limit when you're all stuck in a traffic jam. It can't go faster than the car in front of it. We can accept that reality and decide what else we want to do with our time, like listen to a podcast or sing, or we can stay willful and focused on what is not possible.

Sometimes willingness takes humility, since we have to be willing to acknowledge the reality that we don't know everything. Humility helps healers be patient and listen. I know you've spent tons of time and energy on education and training to become an expert in your field, so in many ways you know things that your clients do not. Yet if you can humble yourself, remembering that you can't know or solve it all, then you might catch sight of something unexpected or let the client have room to find their own way.

Exercise:

As you move through your week, notice the physical and mental signs of willfulness and willingness that come up for you (including any willfulness about doing this exercise).

11. They Don't Want Your Advice (and they don't need it)

11.1 The Importance of Validation

Healing is very, very different from fixing. It's allowing the system, the organism to come to terms with the way things are, and then it rotates. Very often there's change in profound, meaningful ways—ways that no one could tell you about. You have to discover or uncover them yourself through your own willingness to engage.

-Jon Kabat-Zinn

Here's a little experiment. I'm going to tell you some things about my health, and you observe what comes up for you in your body and mind.

I've been living with chronic pain and illness for over 32 years.

As I write this, I have 5 autoimmune diseases, 3 neurological ones, at least 1 gastrointestinal one, and 1 dermatological one.

Some of my diseases are bad enough that I have difficulty doing activities of daily living.

And now I'll add some more information—just notice your reactions:

At the time of most of my diagnoses, I had eaten almost no processed sugar for a year, ate mostly organic and local foods, had tons of vegetables, whole grains, and fruit in my diet, took omega-3 and vitamin D supplements, consumed turmeric regularly, and did not drink caffeine.

At the time of most of my diagnoses, I was going to ecstatic dance 6-8 hours a week, going to Pilates reformer classes twice a week, attending yoga classes 3-4 times a week, and sleeping at least 8 hours a night. In my free time, I enjoyed meditating, kayaking, hiking, and swimming and had lots of social support.

At the time of most of my diagnoses, I was getting massages every other week as well as using a Neti pot, aromatherapy, and dry brushing.

What other information do you find yourself wishing you had? What were your reactions? How are you feeling towards me? What actions do you feel moved to do? What do you feel compelled to say? Are you unconsciously searching for something to blame, for something that I did wrong?

It is really hard for most people to sit with the reality that shit happens. Bodies go haywire. Humans decide to hurt other humans. Sometimes you do "everything right" and shit still happens. There are things that cannot be cured. There are issues in society that are hard to acknowledge. As healers and helpers, people bring these issues to us every day.

At times, what we hear or see may be so shocking that we want to deny that it could happen. Our instinct is to push it away out of fear, to find a way to protect ourselves from it happening to us. That's when we have to be very careful not to blame the victim or client. That's when we have to use all our tools (and consult with other professionals if needed) to be able to validate their experience and allow it into our reality.

The rush to offer unsolicited advice is often our first impulse. It makes us feel helpful, hopeful, like there's something we can do. And it comes from a loving intention.

However, unsolicited advice also means we don't see the person in front of us, that we're failing to hold space for their experience, for their reality. We disempower them by taking a position of knowing better and having that magic fix. Sometimes, like me, they have worked through a lot of pain and grief to come to a place of accepting their situation and working with it rather than against it. The advice-giving sends the receiver through that whole grieving process again, which is exhausting. Advice can also feel like judgment, like a message that the receiver just hasn't tried hard enough, like blaming the victim. Believe me, anyone who's lived with anything chronic (trauma, illness, weight issues, etc.) has tried more things than you can imagine and has likely heard your advice before.

Here's the deal. Shit happens. If you really, truly want to hold space for people, you must come to terms with the suffering that is inherent in life. Just because someone mentions a problem does not mean they're asking for advice. Listen. Wait for people to ask you for help or advice. They might never ask, and that's okay too. Being seen and heard is more valuable than any possible fix. It's part of becoming whole, of healing. One of my teachers, Vanessa Stone, says to remember that healing does not always mean curing. As helpers, we can't cure much, if anything. But we sure as heck can hold a safe space for healing to happen.

Then, if and when clients do come and ask you for advice, there's a much higher probability that they will listen and implement it, and that they will come back to you again in the future, now that you've shown yourself to be a safe person who can hold space for their entire experience. You might well be the only person in their life who is willing and able to do that for them. And that is a priceless gift to your client.

Exercise:

The next time someone brings up a problem with you without immediately asking for input, try listening for at least three minutes without offering advice. You can ask questions to learn more if needed. Then, after at least three minutes of listening, ask them if they'd like to hear a suggestion.

11.2 When People Get Worse

*I have not failed. I've just found 10,000
ways that won't work.*

-*Thomas Edison*

Sometimes, no matter how much space you've held or help you've offered a client, it happens. You've been trying so hard to do all you can, and then they come in and tell you they're feeling worse or they've slipped into old habits.

Naturally, this will affect you. If you're like me, you'll initially either start doubting yourself, get mad, or feel a little hopeless and think about quitting to go bake cupcakes for a living. This is more likely if you've been working with a client for a long time or if they waited a while to tell you they've relapsed.

Being able to predict your reaction to this sort of news can help you prepare. I know that at times, once I hear something like this, one or more of those emotions are on their way. That means I also know to focus on keeping my face caring and listening to the client's story until the initial reflexive responses move through and I feel a little safer to speak.

Clients need to know that we care about them and want to help even when they aren't doing well—especially when they aren't doing well. Shame frequently haunts these situations, so watch carefully for it and see what empathy you can bring to meet it. We all have rough spots and slips. It's part of being human. It's part of healing.

At such times, it's vital to separate behavior from who someone is as a person. Avoid labeling this person as a "resistant client" or a "bad person." Shifting our mental and documentation wording to something like "did not do physical therapy exercises this week" or "used cocaine two times this week" can help both of you stay out of shame and blame, instead shifting to a more productive focus on behavior that can change.

When a client is brave enough to bring their struggles to you, first validate that courage and normalize how challenging change can be. Then listen closely to their tale of what happened. Don't jump to conclusions—sometimes what a client presents as failure is actually a series of small successes that they perceive as not being good enough. Finally, after validation and deep, curious listening, you can go into troubleshooting mode and see what can be done differently in the future. Nothing is wasted, since we can glean as much useful data from failure as we can from success.

Reflection:

What's your initial reaction when a client is struggling? What's your reaction to your own struggles with making changes?

11.3 When People Get Better

*I was so scared to give up depression,
fearing that somehow the worst part of me
was actually all of me.*

-Elizabeth Wurtzel

Now and then comes the moment we've all been waiting for—our client shows improvement. Their symptoms decrease, their pain eases, they do that thing they thought they couldn't do, whatever it is that looks like progress for them. It's lovely. We celebrate with them. We might even tear up a little with shared joy and gratitude.

Here's what many clients don't say. They might not even consciously know it enough to put it into words. Clients often worry that if they get better, we'll abandon them. That we'll kick them out the door at the first sign of positive change. That we'll decide that someone else who is in more pain is more worthy of their appointment time.

And there are other worries that come along with improvement. For some, there's the fear of losing insurance coverage of services, disability payments, or accommodations if they show even a little relief, even though they might well still need the support from those programs.

Others might fear what will be expected of them if they are doing better. They could be imagining being given responsibilities and pressures that they aren't equipped to handle. Or worry that they will no longer be able to rest when they need to, since they won't have their illness as a reason.

The early days of improvement are a delicate time. Like any change, progress will take time to become a habit. Instead of relaxing a little because your client seems able to handle things better on their own now, this is the time to consider giving *more* attention, focusing on areas like relapse prevention strategies, troubleshooting potential challenges, learning to set boundaries, and making statements that leave space for the very human possibility that next week might not be as amazing. There's a bit of a high that can come with feeling better after being miserable. Once that wears off, the real monotonous and unglamorous work of that maintenance stage sets in.

Thus, some of this stage involves holding yourself back from assumptions that it'll be smooth sailing from here on out, some of it is holding the client back from deciding that it'll be smooth sailing from here on out, and some of it is celebrating and realistically looking ahead. Remind clients that this is not the time to quit medications or whatever therapies they have been doing, since those are the things that likely helped them get to this point. In these early days, add supports rather than subtracting them. That'll give your client the best chance for lasting success and address their underlying fears of loss. It may feel like holding back the tides, but it's worth it for sustainable progress.

Reflection:

What are your own fears when a client is making progress? These might include the fear of losing income and having to find a new client.

11.4 It's Going to Be a Little Bumpy

Your clients aren't the only ones making changes. Even by reading this book and implementing the tools, you're also making changes. We have our own reactions to this process.

Bold moves, leaps of faith, whatever you want to call them, are going to stir up our mind's chatter and our parts that want to protect us. They see trying something new as a potential threat to us, and they want to keep us from being hurt. It's part of the deal. Make a big step, the mind runs up and yells for us to back away. Our emotions can get in on it too, namely fear and anxiety.

At times like these, we need to muster the self-compassion to tell ourselves what I once heard a mother say to her son on an Amtrak train. They were standing by the door that led to the next car. On this particular train, the door would slide open at the press of a button, requiring you to cross a short, constantly bouncing and shifting platform before reaching the door to the next car. While crossing, you could hear all the noise from the tracks and feel the wind. The mother knelt down and told her child, "This'll be a bit of an adventure. We're going to go across together. It'll be bumpy, maybe a little loud. Are you ready?" The child took her hand slowly, and they made it across.

Can you be that parent to yourself? To your clients? Are you ready?

If so, let's dive into how to implement these tools.

Reflection:

What's one change you're willing to explore, even if it'll be bumpy?

What's one change you're not yet ready to make?

12. How to Actually Use This Stuff

12.1 Ways to Implement This Stuff

There are so many books out there. Books and workshops and continuing education trainings...so many tools and techniques to learn. We dive into them, come back bright-eyed and inspired, then that high wears off in a week or two as we get busy.

The best way to implement the tools in this book is to use them when you're not at work as well as when you are. The more practice you have with feeling spacious, sitting with emotions and pain without immediately jumping in, and living in line with what's most important to you, the easier it'll be to do it when with your clients. They'll sense it, too.

You may also find other benefits. For example, shame is a critter that can pop up when we're faced with needing to learn something new or try a new technique. Using *Zoom*, the WOE tools, and self-compassion with shame lets us navigate around it and continue our education to become better helpers.

12.2 Helping People You Don't Like

Ever seen two dogs meet and they instantly start snarling at each other? They have no history together, no prior knowledge, but they can't stand being in the same place.

Humans experience that, too. There's no shame in it. No matter how compassionate you are, you will inevitably encounter someone you just don't like.

And, sometimes, that person will be your client.

If a client is threatening emotionally or physically, that is not the time to worry about finding a way to connect with them. Your safety is top priority. Otherwise, assuming that they are safe to be around, here are some ways to cope.

Try to find one thing, no matter how tiny, that you like about them. This could be the color of their shirt, that they were on time for their appointment, that they'll be out of your office in an hour—anything.

> *Be compassionate to everyone. Don't just search for whatever it is that annoys and frightens you, see beyond those things to the basic human being. Especially see the child in the man or woman.*
>
> *-Alice Walker*

Emotions can't be wrong. We will run into clients whose views are widely different from our own. If we focus on the content, it'll feel impossible to connect. Shifting our focus to the common human emotions fosters connection. We all know what it's like to worry about the future, to feel out of control, to feel frustrated or scared. You might not be able to say, "Oh me too!" about whatever they're talking about, but you probably can say, "Wow, it sounds like you're feeling really nervous right now."

Get reflective. Do they remind you of someone in your own life? Do they embody something that you don't like about yourself? Are they reminding you of what you were like before you grew or changed a behavior? Are you jealous of something about them? Are you fearful of something related to their problems or illnesses?

Reflect even more. What biases are you carrying? Some can be sneaky, so look closely. What are you assuming about this person without evidence? What were you taught as a child about people who share characteristics with this one? What are you assuming that they will think about you? Or that they expect of you?

Look at your interactions. Is there something about how you are communicating or the environment that you're in that is affecting your time with this person?

And finally, if you mull over all this stuff and you still just can't *even* with them, it might be time to refer to someone else. There's no shame in that. We are not for everyone, and everyone is not for us. If your primary goal is to be helpful to this person, then referring to someone who is a better fit is still a way of being helpful. Better for both of you that you refer them to someone else rather than you always feeling dread when you see their name on your schedule.

While we're on the topic, there are two kinds of clients who can be particularly challenging: those who have some sort of narcissistic traits and those who tend to reject help.

I'm oversimplifying here, since this isn't a course in psychiatric diagnosis. Put simply, the core of a narcissistic personality structure is incredible insecurity that is so intense that the person can't even be aware of it—in fact, they have to develop a false sense of superiority to avoid feeling any of that insecurity. Their entire personality rallies around them *Truman Show*-style to protect them by creating a version of the world that preserves that inflated self. Anything that might puncture that picture gets spun into being someone else's fault or inadequacy because they cannot acknowledge it as their own. Now combine that with difficulty feeling empathy. This is not an easy way to live, nor is this an easy personality style to live with.

This personality type is not likely to go to therapy or similar healing modalities unless someone has forced them to or there's something they can gain from it. If they do go, they may spend a lot of time picking at the professional's credentials, physical appearance, office, age, and so on. Sometimes these clients spend time educating the professional because they believe they know more than they do.

Other practitioners have a higher probability of encountering this personality for services like massage, acupuncture, and chiropractic care. If you do, one approach is to remain polite but impersonal, not sharing any information that you don't have to, and doing what you can to avoid becoming outwardly agitated (being agitated on the inside is fine). Do your work by the book and document it thoroughly. If they break rules or become dangerous, then of course follow your usual protocols to address the situation.

You may also find yourself in a room with a client who is in great distress, living what they describe as a miserable life.

Your heart breaks for them! Everything in you wants to help them feel better and find solutions. So you start offering assistance. And offering. And offering. Each time, there's a reason it won't work or they've already tried it. You can feel the compassion and life force just seeping out of you. You've given them your best stuff and tried everything! Why can't you get anywhere with them? You might start feeling as hopeless, helpless, and miserable as they are. (This is sometimes referred to as the help-rejecting client.)

What is this client truly wanting? Hint: it's not solutions. What if each time they complain about something, they're really saying, "Can you see me? Can you see how much I'm hurting?" With these clients, validation is most important. Validate their pain to the fullest extent (and maybe even a little more) and let go of expectations of significant change. Maybe they will, maybe they won't, but you continuing to suggest solutions won't get you anywhere but grumpy and drained.

Reflection:

Think of a current client who's been challenging for you. What approaches from this section can you apply to your work with them?

12.3 How to Deal when You're in the Same Boat

I'm writing this book during the 2020 COVID-19 global pandemic. My first day of graduate clinical training as a therapist was 9/11/2001 (because the radio in my 1988 Honda Accord was broken, I didn't know what was happening until I stepped into the rural community mental health center's waiting room right when their TV showed the second plane hitting the tower). In my time as a therapist, there have been numerous distressing, traumatic, and infuriating local, national, and global events that have affected me as well as my clients. At times like these, we and our clients are in the same soup. Moreover, we have very little time to figure out how we are going to cope with it, let alone how to help our clients do it.

Then there are smaller-scale events. I don't know about you, but it's eerie how many times I've had a client come to me with an issue that was really close to what I was dealing with at the time. I never had so many clients struggling with grief at losing their mothers until after my own mother died.

On one hand, we can use our experiences to bolster our empathy and understanding of what these clients might need. On the other hand, we have to increase our caution in these situations to avoid making assumptions or leaning on clients for support that it isn't their job to give.

They're not you. And no matter how similar a situation may sound, it is not *your* situation. Listen closely for the differences. That can help you avoid falling into the assumption trap.

Be vigilant about becoming swept up in your own emotions. Sometimes a client or a case stirs up so much emotion that we can't be effective--and it's wise to recognize when to back away and let someone else step in. Mindfulness practice will also help you sort out what's yours, what's theirs, and when yours is creeping in.

When there's a large-scale event, I try to give myself some time to feel through it before I start seeing clients. This might look like weeping in the shower, stomping around and ranting, scribbling in my journal, curling up in the fetal position in bed, anything that feels right. Once I've had my own raw initial reaction, I'm better able to hold space for whatever reaction my clients may be having. I've made some room.

Whatever the situation, monitor how much you're talking to the client about it—and why you're saying it. Are you sharing something for their direct benefit or your own? Are you trying to prove something? Will this contribute to their treatment, or are you wanting validation and companionship? The more unusual the issue that you have in common with your client, the greater the risk of slipping into oversharing. This temptation is incredibly human, so please be gentle with yourself when you find yourself doing it. Use kindness when keeping yourself accountable.

You and your client might be in the same boat internally rather than externally. Say you have a chronic illness and your client comes in reporting something similar. If what they're describing sounds worse than what you experience with your own illness, you might notice an impulse to distance yourself from the conversation or find flaws in how they're treating their symptoms. Maybe it brings up your fears about what your own disease can do. If they describe something less severe than what you have, or something that you have found a way to overcome, then you might feel an urge to dismiss their issues as not that important or even become annoyed that they're complaining about something that feels minor to you. If they're treating (or not treating) their condition in a different way than you have chosen to do, or have access to resources that you don't, keep an eye out for more powerful reactions. Since so many conditions are common, it's likely you'll come across this situation multiple times in your career and your personal life.

This is also a time to ward off the temptation to assume that you know what the client is experiencing and to dispense advice based on your own experience. Your own lessons learned may very well come in handy, but it'll take more time to determine if and when to share them. Do your best to come to them as a blank slate.

Reflection:

What are some ways that your experience has overlapped with that of a client? How did you deal with it? What would you like to do differently in the future?

12.4 Tragedy in a Fishbowl

Being at work doesn't protect us from life events. Death, injury, natural disaster, interpersonal violence can all follow us in the door no matter how many badges and keys we use.

These things are hard enough to deal with without the added pressure of all eyes being on us as we try to find our way. Tragedy in a helping role brings:

Logistical decisions: How to keep track of clients, how to contact them if they need to be informed, how to make sure that they can access the care they need and triage that care if resources are scarce, how to assign staff duties in the most efficient and useful way, making decisions about leave policies.

Tending to client and other stakeholder concerns: Finding clear and calm messaging about what has happened and what will happen, offering reassurance, holding space to hear their feelings and questions, being a steady and compassionate presence.

Dealing with outside entities (possibly): Deciding about press releases or whether to talk with the media, managing image, dealing with any investigative bodies, making reports if needed to police or other agencies, consulting with legal counsel and liability insurance.

(For management/supervisors): Supporting staff, creating room for them to debrief, checking in to see what is needed, offering food, drink, and quiet spaces to rest and grieve, bringing in outside support like counselors as needed, reminding staff of EAP options if available.

Personal needs: Figuring out own personal needs, activating personal support networks, determining when able to work and when to take time off, processing events (including own reactions to clients' reactions).

It's a LOT.

I know. I've been there. While working at a huge agency in very busy mental health clinics, I twice had to deal with unexpectedly losing coworkers. Once was to a car accident on the way to work, and another was due to a completely unforeseen situation. Both times we found out in the morning once we were already at work and their first clients of the day were sitting in the waiting room. There was so little time to process our own shock and dismay before having to compose ourselves enough to give our clients the news.

Do you tell clients what happened? Do you tell them how you're feeling? There are so many schools of thought on disclosure. I lean towards the advice that a colleague gave me when I started my first job as a psychologist: "Be honest." Being honest doesn't mean that you say everything that goes through your head. To me, it means you don't pretend that everything is fine when you and your client have just found out that their doctor (and your colleague) died mere hours earlier. That you don't have to be a blank-faced robot.

The fine line here is that we have to remember that our clients are NOT here to be our support system. Watch carefully for slipping into long monologues about what you're thinking or feeling. If you disclose something, keep it short and sweet and think about whether it's relevant to their care. Clients aren't our captive audience.

Here's an example:

Too Much: Can you believe this happened? I'm so upset about it. I'm having trouble sleeping, and I'm eating ice cream all the time...I feel like it's my fault somehow. And I really regret the time I told them that I couldn't help out because I was too busy. I haven't been a good friend to them or other people lately, which my therapist says could be because of how my mother was....

Just Enough: You're right, it's really surreal and sad that this happened. I still can't quite believe it myself. Tragedies like this can really get us looking at our lives and what's important to us. Has that been happening with you lately? How have you been coping with it?

12.5 You Have the Power

Now that we've covered scenarios where we feel helpless, let's turn to ways that we have significant influence.

You're freakin' powerful. You really are. Powerful to have gotten this far, powerful in the healing work you do, and powerful to your clients. Yep. You have a lot of power in that relationship. Even when you don't feel like it.

When someone comes to a healer/helper, they are engaging in a vulnerable act. They are admitting that they need something from you. That they can't do it by themselves. That they are struggling. Your clients will tell you things that they don't tell anyone else, things that they've never spoken aloud. If you work hands-on with bodies or lead them in physical movement, that's an additional type of power since your client is literally putting themselves in your hands and trusting that you won't injure them.

The power also dwells in the one-way street of the situation. You know much more about your client than they do about you—which is as it should be in order for you to be helpful. However, this dynamic also keeps you in a power-up position.

Now that you know you have this power, you also need to know that all of your words, advice, and actions are amplified in your client's mind. Choose them with caution. Be wary of your wording. Suggestions are better than commands, although they may still hear your suggestion as a command.

The same goes for any stumble in the relationship. If you put your foot in your mouth or make a mistake, do what you can to admit it, apologize, and make repairs. If you don't, your client might vanish and possibly avoid seeking help from anyone in your profession.

And, obviously, avoid going into the romantic or sexual realm with your clients, especially while they are actively under your care and/or if they are likely to want to return to see you after they leave your care. There's a ton written about this and ensconced in ethical standards and laws, for good reason. The imbalance of power makes it impossible for a client to make a truly free decision.

My first clinical supervisor gave me a mug as a parting gift at the end of my time with her. I used to be puzzled by the Maya Angelou quote engraved on its gently curving side:

Only equals can be friends

. I couldn't figure out why she chose that quote of all the quotes out there. I knew the ways it can apply to inequality and racial injustice, but it took more years of clinical training, anti-racism education, and some experiences with academic politics to realize the wisdom in her reminder that these imbalances in power prevent true, freely chosen relationships. I can't be a genuine friend with a client because I'll always have the power of deep knowledge about them and their vulnerability with me. I can't be a true friend with someone like a boss who has to evaluate my work performance because they'll have that power over me, which will influence whether I feel like I can set boundaries or give them honest feedback. It might even affect the kinds of activities I would agree to do with them or what I would share with them.

Only equals can be friends. You don't have to be someone's friend to help them. And don't rely on your clients, staff, or supervisees for friendship and socialization. They are not your built-in family. It's convenient, but not healthy. Yet another reason to build a life outside of your work.

A special note about supervisees, interns, and trainees: You might want to give them a realistic view of the field you're in and the challenges you face, but keep a filter on it. There's a power differential here, and they didn't sign up to be your confidant or the person you vent to about every frustration or policy change. If you do that, it's a little like putting a child in the position of listening to a parent talk about problems in the marriage. They're unprepared for it, they don't have any power to change any of it, it unfairly asks them to choose a side, and it detracts from what they are there to do.

Watch out for this same temptation if you run any kind of support group, therapy group, or teach a class. Since they are sharing, it can be tempting to share as well. And hey, having an audience can feel pretty nice. But watch closely, since this can slide into taking the time and focus away from the group members or students. Guard against this temptation even more at times when you're having issues with the agency or studio, since it can start seeming like a good idea to get the group on your side and maybe even suggest an action they can take. They aren't your minions, so be very aware of that power differential thing here.

This is a simplistic slice of a deeply complex pie. I've focused on roles, but keep in mind that race, gender, sexuality, disability, age, citizenship status, socioeconomic status, neurodiversity, and other factors intersect to affect power dynamics more than I have space to discuss here.

Exploration:

What are the power dynamics in your professional life? Where do you have influence? Who has power over you?

12.6 Case Examples

Let's take a look at a few fictional case examples and see how we can apply what we've learned so far.

A client comes to an integrated health clinic to deal with a long list of chronic health issues. A month into his treatment there, his nutritionist and acupuncturist run into each other in the staff kitchen. The nutritionist asks the acupuncturist if they've had any progress with this client, since she has not been able to see any change, just resistance and lack of energy. Surprised, the acupuncturist describes him as an engaged and improving client.

The nutritionist can't understand—she has been giving the client excellent information, created a detailed meal plan for him, and spends their entire appointment time educating him. The acupuncturist, on the other hand, had spent a large part of their early sessions interviewing the client about the history of his health issues and validating how difficult it can be to live with them. The acupuncturist has experienced the client as motivated and willing to try the exercises and herbs that they've prescribed.

Why the difference?

A client comes in and shares a story full of grief and loss, along with many physical symptoms. They are weepy and sometimes even unable to talk because of crying. Their story is heartbreaking to hear. The therapist immediately hands them the tissue box as soon as they start crying. Client continues to cry, almost wailing, on and on. The therapist shifts in their chair frequently and finds that they have some tears starting to roll down their own cheeks. The client hasn't said any coherent words for many minutes. The therapist keeps saying "it's okay" over and over, asking questions about what's wrong in an effort to get the client to talk.

A client comes in and shares that something horrific has just happened, and the practitioner says, "That's terrible! I'm so sorry. How did you do with following your nutrition plan for the week?"

A client comes in sharing that their car was stolen the previous night. The practitioner tells a detailed story about how their own car was stolen 10 years ago and what they did in that situation.

What do you see in these examples? What's happening?

The client comes in for an initial session, and everything she says fits with the therapist's experience. The therapist has seen dozens of people with the same issues and has found that certain techniques work well. About 10 minutes in, the therapist says, "I know exactly what you're talking about! Here's what you need to do..." and generously proceeds to share all their best advice for the rest of the appointment. At the end of the session, the therapist feels glowy and competent. The client thanks the therapist and says that they'll reach out to schedule when they know their availability. The therapist feels helpful...until they realize that weeks have gone by and the client hasn't contacted them to schedule another appointment.

What happened?

13. Planning for the Long Haul

13.1 Sustainability

Compassionate people ask for what they need. They say no when they need to, and when they say yes, they mean it. They're compassionate because their boundaries keep them out of resentment.

-Brené Brown, Rising Strong

We've talked about mindsets, coping skills, and other ways to help you be a more sustainable healer and helper. The next sections will expand on the practice aspects of a sustainable helping career.

When taking on a role, imagine yourself in it in a year, three years, ten years from now. What do you foresee hating about it? Can you identify anything that will wear you down or burn you out? See what you can adjust or put into place now to help address those things proactively. Or set a date on which you promise yourself you'll reevaluate and leave the role if needed.

If you've already been in the role for a while, what can you do now to make it more comfortable? And do you want to stay in it as it is now? Is it worth trying to make the changes necessary to improve it?

Some behaviors are inherently unsustainable in the long run, such as:

➤ Working so many hours a week that you cannot have a social life or take care of basic needs like medical appointments, laundry, or meals.

➤ Working without at least one day off a week (unless it is a schedule where you get a sizeable chunk of time off on a routine basis, like 10 days on, 7 days off).

➤ Working for 6 months or a year without taking any time off.

➤ Providing physical healing modalities like massage to the point of injury with no healing/rest time.

➤ Working without eating or getting adequate hydration regularly

➤ Setting fees or bartering at rates that don't allow you to cover your own expenses and needs.

(I know these situations are an inherent part of many people's working lives as they try to survive in the face of vast income inequality and abusive labor practices. In this section, I'm speaking to those of us who have the privilege to be able to choose how we work. If you're lucky enough to have a choice, then choose something sustainable.)

We all have those days or weeks that are just extra hectic. That's not what I'm talking about here. I'm talking about when these behaviors continue for months or years.

We are professionals. Our instruments? Our minds, bodies, and hearts. Like Olympic athletes or other professionals, we need a certain level of care and attention to our well-being in order to perform our best. Sure, we can treat ourselves like the equivalent of a partying rock star, staying up too late, working too many days in a row, giving too much of ourselves, but unless we have the luck to have the invincibility of Mick Jagger, we won't last long. And even if we physically endure, we'll be drained on the inside.

When I took a restorative yoga teacher training with Judith Hanson Lasater, she told us, "Never live at the edge of your time, energy, or money." Not always possible, but a worthy goal indeed.

Sustainability can extend beyond how you do your work to include the type of work you do. While it's important to hone your skills and practice your craft, you don't have to keep doing it exactly the same way for your entire career. For example, my former supervisor always claimed that you can do seven years of full-time trauma work and then something has to change. Seven years was the limit. Sometimes we can think that that changing is chickening out, that we're being wishy-washy or fickle or uncommitted. Please remember that your helping and healing career is allowed to morph and grow with you.

When you first start out, you might do full-time hands-on face-to-face work with clients in direct service. As years go by, you might add teaching, supervising, or consulting. Or you might do part-time helping work and develop another form of income. That form of income could be directly related to your profession, such as public speaking, teaching workshops, or writing books about your field to things like real estate, selling arts or crafts, or waiting tables if that gives you a break and helps you recharge.

Listening to Elizabeth Gilbert's *Magic Lessons* podcast (episode 201) reminded me that many of us carry the misconception that service work has to be serious, maybe even that it has to be a painful sacrifice. Think of all the artists, musicians, comedians, writers, cartoonists, and other people who have made a difference in your life...they are healers and helpers in their own way. As I write this during the COVID-19 pandemic, artistic creations are giving people safe options for much-needed distraction, hope, adventure, connection, and relaxation. If you are being moved to follow a path that seems "silly" or "not serious enough," reflect on how people who are lit up inside help others heal, no matter what work they're doing.

We are not our jobs. At the same time, see how you can bring more "you" into your workday. The more fully we can be ourselves wherever we go, the less drained we'll feel. (I also know that unfortunately at this time, discrimination and -isms mean that sometimes we have to downplay parts of ourselves for safety or other reasons.) You may have to bring in parts of yourself on the sly, like listening to your favorite music or podcasts on headphones or in the car, wearing meaningful jewelry under your clothes, and so on.

I also want to note that "full-time client work" does NOT mean seeing clients face-to-face or hands-on for 40 hours a week. There may be a few modalities where that is doable, but it isn't realistic in most kinds of helping work. Each client, each session is accompanied by some kind of administrative work. You may also have to consult with other practitioners,

THEY'RE NOT BROKEN · 123

do some research, get supplies, change sheets, clean up—not to mention recharge yourself and tend to your body.

There's changing the things that we work with, and then there's also changing the way that we do things. That takes some willingness and humility. For example, while writing this book, I have been dealing with flares of psoriatic arthritis that are affecting my hands for the first time. I'm someone who has always loved writing by hand in a beautiful journal or on a legal pad, or at the very least typing on a computer. It took me a long time to finally try dictation because it didn't seem like "real writing" to me. I found the *Dragon Naturally Speaking* software, I bought a book by Scott Baker with the nifty title *Training Your Dragon*, I got a good headset and a quality voice recorder, and now I'm learning a whole new way of writing that uses my brain in a different way and is in some ways more efficient. I have more options for how to write, which makes me more sustainable.

Because of the global pandemic, I have also shifted to offering 100% telehealth services right now. And that has also made me more sustainable because I'm able to focus on seeing my clients instead of all the other things that can be very painful or difficult to do, like driving and walking into an office building and arranging chairs. I have a very comfy armchair at home. I have lots of blankets and fluffy socks and heating pads and all the things I need to be as comfortable as I can be given the situation. In some ways, I'm providing better services because I'm focused on the essence of my work. Disability has forced me to boil things down to the very essential core.

Exercise:

How about for you? What's the most essential part of the work that you want to be doing or that you need to be doing? What lies at the heart of it? And how many different ways can you do that same work? Do you still want to be doing it the way that you're doing it now? We're allowed to change and grow, just like our clients are. Let yourself dream a little. Let yourself play a little.

13.2 Self-Care

You can have it all. You just can't have it all at once.

-Oprah Winfrey

What are your non-negotiable self-care needs? Do you even know?

Self-care often isn't bubble baths and napping in hammocks (although those can be lovely). Self-care is usually a little boring or even scary, like looking at bank accounts, getting medical tests, and setting boundaries with others. Doesn't make for a pretty social media photo, but it can foster greater peace of mind and better physical and financial health. If you own your own healing practice as a business, then self-care extends to taking care of your business affairs. So unglamorous, I know.

Areas of self-care:
➢ Physical
➢ Emotional

➤ Intellectual
➤ Relationships
➤ Financial/Material
➤ Administrative (like renewing driver's license, etc.)
➤ Environment around you
➤ Spiritual (for some people)

If you own a business, then many of these categories will have both a personal and a business version, such as doing your household budget and your business profit-and-loss statements. Professional training can be self-care since it often provides connection with others in your field, a break from direct client contact, and the confidence that can come with additional practice and skills. Training can't be your only form of self-care, though, and watch out for the temptation to escape into endless trainings and certifications as a way to try to counteract impostor syndrome.

Exercise:

How well do you know your own rhythms? If you can't answer these right now, start observing yourself as you go through your week and see what you can learn about your natural preferences.

1.   Best time of day/day of the week to focus?

2.   Best time of day/day of the week to work with others?

3.   Best time of day/day of the week for physical activity or tasks that take little mental energy?

4.   Best environment for work (sound vs. silent, etc.)

5. What do you need in order to work well (good food, movement, comfy clothes, etc.)?

6. What factors make it difficult for you to do good work?

7. How much recovery time do you need after each meeting or session? Each day? Each week?

8. What tasks annoy or drain you the most?

9. What tasks soothe or recharge you?

10. What kind of colleagues do you enjoy? What kind of clients?

11. What kind of colleagues are challenging for you? What kind of clients?

Exercise:

Take 5 minutes and list all the "parts" of yourself you can. These can be roles you play, activities you enjoy, needs that you have.

Which parts on the list get a lot of attention? Which have been neglected? How can you scoop up and nourish the neglected pieces, even in a small way? How can you remind yourself of all that you are beyond what you can give others? Make a plan.

For example, if "world traveler" shows up on your list, but travel is not possible for you right now, perhaps you can find some pictures of distant places to have around you in your office or watch some travel shows during your downtime. You could plan hypothetical trips, research hotels and sights to see, go someplace in your town you've never been, try foods from a different culture, or watch videos on how best to pack a suitcase.

13.3 Self-Compassion

Sure, you say, this self-care thing sounds great, but how am I ever going to get anything done?

Self-compassion can be an excellent tool for finding balance, if used in the right way. Here are three common mistakes and misconceptions about self-compassion. Your clients might be doing these as well, so they're good to know.

Mistake One: Letting Yourself Waaaaay off the Hook

It's not necessarily self-compassionate to let ourselves blow off all responsibility for extended periods of time. It's not necessarily self-compassionate to eat foods that make our bodies feel ill. Or to avoid those phone calls or emails that have an effect on our future selves, like dealing with insurance or student loans. True self-compassion finds the balance between rest and the less fun activities that are important for deep self-care on a practical level. We keep ourselves accountable and ask for support when needed.

Mistake Two: Avoiding Taking Responsibility

Compassion and empathy help us understand where someone is coming from when they do or say something. We can see things from their perspective and how they may have decided to act in a certain way. However, this is different from saying that they aren't responsible for their actions. We can understand the reasons without the reasons becoming excuses.

Now let's turn this idea towards ourselves. If we habitually avoid taking responsibility for our choices and actions, that's not self-compassion. Avoiding responsibility also means avoiding the opportunity to grow and do better next time. We can explore our reasons, triggers, and motivations with curiosity—being careful not to use them as excuses. Think of an excuse as giving up on yourself. It's not empowering. It's saying that you can't possibly change. (And we know that isn't true. You wouldn't be reading this if at least some part of you wasn't curious about how to make your life and the lives of others different in some way.)

Mistake Three: Giving up Too Soon

Anything new takes time. I'm going to repeat that: Anything new takes time. Most of us weren't taught self-compassion, so this is new stuff. It's going to take more than a day, a week, maybe more than a year to adopt a more self-compassionate attitude. Plus, we're working with minds that are geared for survival, hanging onto painful memories and ditching the pleasant ones. We're going uphill in the snow both ways, y'all. As mentioned earlier, our minds will kick up a fuss. That's to be expected when we make any kind of change. Eventually it'll settle into a new groove.

A note to anyone who was labeled a "gifted child" or got through school with little effort: you're not going to be able to do everything well on the first try. I know that was your experience for much of your early life (it was mine too), but at some point you're going to run into something that takes a little more effort and time. That doesn't mean that there's anything wrong with you! It's just how the world works. If you can meet that challenge with curiosity instead of anger or helplessness, you'll get even stronger. Plus, it gets boring if everything is easy, like those video games that you can beat in a day. Challenge helps us build our muscles of persistence and courage. I hope you can take advantage of those opportunities.

13.4 Connection

It is as if when we are "in session" we cease to exist in the outside world. What are the effects of this compartmentalized isolation?...we also may become secretive, mysterious, aloof, and evasive when we are not at work, while we continue to struggle to be authentic, transparent, and genuine with clients. We retreat inside ourselves for comfort and pat ourselves on the back for being so professional.

-Jeffrey Kottler, On Being a Therapist

Friendships

You probably feel like you connect with people all the time, especially if you use a modality that involves talking with clients. We have to remind ourselves that as deep and meaningful as our connections with clients can be, we still need our own personal relationships with non-clients. (My fellow introverts might groan at the idea of spending time with even more people. I'll reassure you by saying that it doesn't have to be every day or for long stretches of time—it just has to be a regular part of your life.)

Now if you recall the beginning of this book, you'll re-member my description of lots of people in my personal life treating me like their own private crisis hotline. People are probably drawn to you because of your caring and compassionate nature. So we have to remember that in our personal lives, relationships need to be a relatively equal two-way street.

Check in with yourself. Are you sharing as much as you're listening? Are your conversations often about things other than deep trauma or solving the other person's problems? How do you feel when you leave the interaction? Energized? Drained? Like you spent the afternoon at work? Resentful? Do you feel you can express yourself without walking on eggshells? We all take care of each other sometimes, but if caretaking is the only way you interact, look carefully at that friendship. You might have taken on a "client" without realizing it.

Friendships also differ from client relationships in that we have even more right to decide we don't want to pursue them. You've probably had clients whom you wouldn't choose spend time with if they weren't clients, but you can make it work. Remember, friendships are different. We can be selective. And we don't have to have an elaborate reason for not wanting to hang out with someone. They don't have to be labeled an energy vampire or anything like that. You can set boundaries based solely on preferences rather than protection. For real. Your time and energy is precious, so spend it where you want to rather than where you think you have to in order to be polite or nice.

Having friendships can also be protective. Without people in our personal lives to talk to and connect with, we risk gradually crossing lines with our clients. It can become tempting to disclose too much, to become loose about enforcing boundaries, to share our own struggles in detail, or even to want to invite them to spend time together outside the office. (Rules about this sort of behavior and relationships with clients vary from profession to profession, of course. Make sure to know yours.) In general, the more of a whole person you can be outside of work, the better a helper you can be to your client because you won't be tempted to use them to meet your own needs.

Networking

Did you just cringe at the word "networking"? Many healers and helpers do—you're not unusual. The word carries a slightly slimy feel for some people, and the idea of talking to strangers terrifies or exhausts others.

Have you ever run into someone else who does what you do, perhaps at a training or conference, and you walk away from the conversation feeling uplifted and inspired? Have their business card in your pocket or their contact information in your phone, or at least know where they work? Surprise! You just networked. Now you have someone to consult and refer to, someone who might keep you in mind if an opportunity arises.

Or you meet a colleague through another colleague? Yep, networking!

Think of networking as building a beautiful web of fellow healers and helpers who know and support each other, each sharing their particular skills. Networking is what you do all the time anyway: building rapport and learning about someone. You meet new people each time you get a new client, so we know you know how to do that part. It's just happening in a different setting (or online).

Networking can be one way that helpers help one another. None of us have all the skills and knowledge that we need, but together we just might. Think of it as a group private practice on a global scale. For example, I am absolutely no good at working with children. I don't have training in it, I don't have experience in it, and it doesn't fit my skill set. When someone reaches out to me asking for help with a child, I need to have people in my web who can do this work.

Consultation and Other Forms of Support

When I was in graduate school, I heard "consult, consult, consult" over and over. Not sure what to do with a client? Consult with a colleague or supervisor. Having an emotional response to a session? Consult. Facing a sticky ethical issue? Consult. Client presenting an issue you know little about? Consult.

Consultation was easy when I worked in agencies where a fellow therapist was literally on the other side of the wall. In private practice, it takes more effort to find consultation, particularly if you're the only person there or the only one who practices your modality.

Depending on your modality, you may be able to find consultation groups through professional organizations, Facebook groups, or listservs. You can also make your own and spread the word. If you'd rather keep it small, make yourself a list of colleagues you know who might be willing to consult one-on-one.

Negotiate the terms of the consultation as well. Some people are happy to consult for free, especially if it is brief. Some consultation groups are free; others may charge dues. If you are needing in-depth consultation about a topic, you may need to offer compensation to an expert in that area. If you are consulting a person from a marginalized group about how to work with people from that group or other diversity issues, compensation is very important because of the amount of emotional and professional labor involved.

These kinds of relationships don't have to be about clinical issues. Perhaps you know several other practitioners who want to work on similar business goals. You can create your own support group to encourage each other and share information. For example, the group could pick a business or marketing book to read together and spend some time discussing and coworking on projects based on the suggestions in the book.

Even if you don't talk while coworking, setting aside a chunk of time to come together and work on your to-do list is powerful. This can happen over video chat or in person. Need emotional support while putting together your tax information? The group can be there. Been procrastinating writing your newsletter? The group can be there. Have an idea for a new healing offering, but aren't sure how to describe it in your marketing? The group can be there. Celebrating a successful month? The group can be there.

The truth is, this work we do can be lonely. Because of our commitment to honoring the trust clients put in us, we carry client information and experiences that we can't share with many people. In fact, the more intense and traumatic the material that we witness is, the less likely we are to be able to say anything about it. Depending on your line of work, you might not be able to give much of an answer when asked, "How was your day?" We often go from the warm camaraderie of our training programs to standing on what feels like our own in an overwhelming new world. The good news? We also have the potential and skills to deeply support each other.

Something Else

When we're in the weeds and slogging through our days, all we can see is the to-do list in front of us. Our world gets really small. Zooming out to connect with something beyond the day's agenda can energize and support us in our work. This something can be a sense of greater purpose, ancestors (relatives and/or people who have done the kind of work you do in the past), spiritual beliefs, nature...anything that feels expansive to you. Remember that you can connect with nature no matter where you are, since we ARE nature. Nature is the dust mites in a tall office building as well as the lush grounds of a wooded retreat center. The client before you is nature, the sun and breeze in a parking lot, the water in your glass.

Exercises:

Make two lists: one of people in your professional life, and one of people in your personal life. (It's okay if one or both of them are very short.) Looking at the lists, what support do you already have? What kinds of connections and support would you like more of? Which existing connections would you like to nurture?

Now make a separate list of things you like to do and places you like to spend time, even if you have never done them or haven't done them in a long time. This list can be your starting point for finding more people and/or growing the relationships you already have. For example, if you love hiking and hate bars, then skip the networking happy hour and see if any of your colleagues would like to go for a hike or have a picnic.

If you like, find some way to remind yourself of connection to something greater. It might be something you wear, something you put in your workspace, a quote or mantra, a little ritual at the start of your day, anything that helps you feel yourself as part of a bigger picture.

13.5 Boundaries

We hear a lot about self-care, or at least about what kinds of activities we should be doing. We hear less about how to actually make that happen in our lives. The best self-care plan in the world can be rendered useless if we don't know how to do one thing: set boundaries.

I know you know how to carve out space for your clients. You make a spot on your calendar for an appointment. You gently close the office door, or silence your phone, or smooth out the sheets on the massage table, or pull the curtain around the exam table, or create an energetic protective circle...all the ways you physically, mentally, and energetically make a bubble so you can focus on the work at hand.

I'm proposing that you set that skill to work for yourself as well. It'll feel awkward, selfish, and unnecessary at first, and now you know how to sit with emotions and remember how you have space for all those feelings and more. Your mind may spew commentary—and now you know how to get un-stuck from those thoughts. Consider it an experiment. Try taking small steps towards meeting your needs and see what happens.

I will note that any experiment worth its salt needs more than one data point, so please keep taking steps. Many years ago, when I was overloaded and doing a terrible job of self-care, my acupuncturist told me that I needed to show my nervous system that I could take a break and the world wouldn't crumble. The next day, I decided to try taking fifteen minutes to put my legs up the wall and listen to peaceful music. Halfway through my rest break, my partner at the time had a medical emergency (that turned out okay). It took me a while to get up the nerve to try taking a break again after that, since it felt like solid proof that everything was resting on my very tense shoulders and I had to be ever-vigilant. With time and repetition, I've been able to get more data points, more breaks that did not correlate with a crisis ensuing, and my nervous system is learning that rest can be okay.

If you've had people run over your boundaries in the past, you might find yourself bracing for conflict when you start setting boundaries around your self-care, even if no one is giving you a hard time about doing so. That can calm down with time and practice as well.

Now, some people will push against your boundaries, especially if you haven't historically set or enforced them. Imagine you are standing in front of a vending machine. You put in your money and push the button for the snack you want. Nothing happens, no snack. What's the first thing you do? Probably push the button again, right? Still no snack. You push the button again, maybe give the machine a smack. Some people even shake the machine. But eventually, if there's no result, you walk away. You realize it's not going to give you what you expected to get.

That's how it works when we first start setting boundaries with people in our lives. They're used to us doing a certain thing when they push our buttons. If they don't get that response, then they push the button more and more. If we can hold firm to our new boundary, they finally realize that we're not going to do what they want and stop pushing. Behavioral psychology calls the increased button pushing an extinction burst. When we don't get the expected result from an action, we do more of that action until we eventually give up. If you don't know about extinction bursts, it can feel like you've made things worse by setting the boundary, but it's really a sign that the other person is noticing the change. Hang in there (unless the situation is abusive or dangerous in other ways, then do what you need to for safety).

Reflection:

What's one specific boundary you can set to protect your self-care and be more sustainable?

13.6 Accountability

One of the reasons our clients come to us is accountability. When we're wanting to make changes, it's useful to be able to report our progress to someone and get help to navigate obstacles.

Can you identify someone in your life who can be an accountability partner for the changes you want to make? This can be as simple as dropping a text or an email when you complete an action or a more elaborate recurring check-in meeting. Or perhaps you do activities together, like a gym buddy or someone who'll meditate with you in the conference room at lunch. If you can't find a buddy in person, there are some habit tracking apps and social media communities out there that might be a fit. I've even found that something as simple as sheets of stickers and a wall calendar can be a simple and effective tracking system. (But then again, I love stickers.)

Your accountability goals don't need to be as formal as a treatment plan. Just make sure you start small, realistic, and specific. Saying "practice better self-care" is meaningless. Saying "leave work on time 2 days a week" is meaningful. See what small steps can give you the most for your efforts. If you're having trouble identifying some, try looking at any physical or social needs that aren't being met right now. Getting enough sleep, water, or food in a day has a powerful trickle-down effect.

Exercise:

Identify 2-3 goals and brainstorm ways to keep yourself accountable as you work towards them.

13.7 Remember Your Why

*To get to the values underlying a goal, you
need to ask yourself, "What's this goal in
the service of? What will it enable me to
do that's truly meaningful?"*

-Russ Harris

Helpers and healers do all kinds of work that other people
would shrink away from. And why? Why do you listen to the
horrific stories, spend your days up to your elbows in massage
oil and laundry, visit filthy homes, roll over and answer the
phone in the middle of deep sleep because you're on call, learn
about clients' digestive output in intense detail, clean bodies,
or whatever it is that you do? Why? Why do you show up
even on days you don't feel motivated? (Motivation isn't re-
quired for action, by the way. But you knew that already.)

Probably because there's something really important about
it for you. Probably because doing this work helps move you
closer to the kind of person you want to be. (If that's not true,
it's okay. Although you might want to think about why you're
here.)

Let's get some clarity on this why. That can help pull you
through some tough times and guide your choices. Just to be
clear, this why goes beyond paying the bills.

This why runs deep, down to the heart of who you want to
be in the world and what you want your life to mean. This
why isn't a goal, like "because I want to cure cancer" or "because I want to feed hungry families." Those are goals with
measurable outcomes.

The bigger why has no end point. This why is made up of qualities that you want to embody, that you would want on your personal mission statement or motto, that are your mantra. Qualities can be lived but never completely achieved.

Living in a way that reflects one's values is not just about what you do, it is also about how you do things.

- Deborah Day

Here's another way to look at it. You can travel east, right? And as you go east, you'll encounter places like New Orleans, India, Japan. But you can never get to East itself. Qualities are like East, and goals are like those places along the way. You'll never get to East, much like you can never be done being an honest person or a dependable person.

That may sound disheartening, but it's actually freeing. It means you have your whole life to be guided by these principles. They'll always be with you, and you can't fail since you can always try again in the next moment to make a choice that moves you towards them. They're infinite.

What are these principles? Sorry, I can't tell you. They're yours. There are no right or wrong ones. But they have to be about you—we can't set them for other people or control other people's behavior. So you can value the quality of being caring, but winning the Nobel Peace Prize can't be one of the qualities since that is 1) a goal and 2) involves other people doing things.

Exercise:

I invite you to take a little time with this and think about 3-5 principles or qualities that are most important to you. If you're getting hung up on what you think they "should" be because of what you've been taught by family or religion or culture, list those to get them out of the way, then make a list of the ones you truly value.

If you're getting stuck, imagine that you're at your 100th birthday party and people from various areas of your life are making speeches about you. How would you like them to describe you? How would you like to describe yourself and how you behaved in your life?

Once you identify them, sit with them for a little while and see how they feel in your body. Adjust your list as needed until they feel right.

Find a way to remind yourself of them. This could be a list on your phone's lock screen, a collage, a sticky note, a song, a voice memo, you name it.

And now take them out for a test drive! Pick one to focus on for the day or the week and see if you can infuse it into your behavior and choices for that time period. For example, if you chose dependable as one of your qualities, you can wait in line dependably, answer phone calls dependably, do just about anything dependably. If you're familiar with setting intentions, it's the same idea. It's not going to magically cure burnout, but operating based on what's most important to us can be part of preventing burnout and maintaining connection with our clients and our work.

13.8 If You Work in an Agency...

I have so much paperwork. I'm afraid my paperwork has paperwork.

-Gabrielle Zevin

Clearly your options for setting up your schedule and who you see, where you work, and so on won't be as plentiful when working in an agency or someone else's practice. However, you might be able to improve your situation through actions like these.

Identify mutually beneficial swaps. Find colleagues who are burned out on some tasks that you would prefer to be doing, and propose a temporary or permanent trade, if your supervisors agree.

If you can't reduce your hours, see if you can vary the ways you spend those hours (rote tasks like copying, tidying, or filing vs. direct contact hours vs. paperwork).

Always frame your suggestions in ways that show how they will benefit the agency. Of course staff morale is important, but administration won't usually make a change simply because the staff is tired or overwhelmed by a situation. There's a better chance of success (although never guaranteed) if you can explain how a change will reduce costs, take less time and free up staff to do other more lucrative activities, improve public relations/standing with the community or stakeholders, reduce expensive errors, decrease the risk of being sued, increase quality of care and client satisfaction, be more compliant with regulations, make the most of existing resources—things like that. Listen closely when the administrators talk and speak to them in their language so they can hear you.

Explore all the resources available to you. Is there an ergonomics consultant you didn't know existed? Or a room of unused furniture so you can exchange your chair for one that doesn't have a stuck wheel? If your workspace is uncomfortably cold, maybe you have an officemate who is burning up in their spot and would be happy to trade. If you're lucky and have benefits through your job, do they happen to include an employee assistance program for free counseling sessions, coverage for massage or chiropractors, discounts for meal kits or exercise facilities, or a wellness program?

Sometimes, depending on your field, you might be able to ask for flexible hours, more time off, specific duties, or other perks in lieu of pay increases. Those are more feasible under tight budgets.

If your agency can't offer you anything in terms of support, look at what you can control. Is it time for a comfier pair of shoes so your feet don't ache from a long day of hard hospital floors? Is it possible to bring in a few personal items for your desk or vehicle to make you smile or bring you comfort? I'm personally very selective about the mugs I use at work...I need them to have a comforting shape and weight as well as interesting textures to run my fingers over to help ground me during intense sessions. Maybe there's a five-minute guided breathing exercise you can listen to on your phone during your workday or a coworker to swap a funny story with each afternoon.

Finally, if you can't change anything at all in your work situation, think about what you can do before and after work to ease your stress and recharge. This could require some serious soul-searching to determine what is truly essential and what activities can be set aside for the time being. It could be small steps like making sure to eat breakfast, deciding to sing along to your favorite music on the way to work instead of listening to the news, calling a non-work friend during lunch, or asking your household to leave you alone for 15 minutes when you first get home.

Exercise:

If you work in an agency, what are 3 suggestions from this chapter that you could try? When and how could you try them?

13.9 What to Consider When Taking on New Clients and Roles

I'm going to speak here to those of you who can choose which clients you work with. I know if you're in an agency, spa, studio, or someone else's practice, you might have to work with whoever they want you to see.

You have a big heart and want to help as many people as possible, right? You believe strongly in the techniques you use. Besides, you could use the income. So why not say yes to every potential client who comes calling?

Because every yes is also a no. Every yes means you're saying no to another potential client, to an hour or more of your own time, to other opportunities. Depending on the type of work you do, you might be saying yes to this client for months or even years.

Our helping work starts with that first contact from a client. Sometimes the most healing thing we can offer is a solid list of referrals to other professionals who will be a better fit. Early in your practice, you might be tempted to take on any client you can get. You might feel terrified to send one off to someone else. I promise, your future self will thank you. We are in a relationship with our clients, and we need to be as thoughtful about entering into these relationships as we are with other types of relationships in our lives.

Here are some questions to ask yourself when you're making these decisions:

Timing: Do I reasonably have space to take on this client at this time? Does my current schedule have an open time that fits their availability? Is taking on this client going to mean that I skip lunch, come in extra early, stay late, miss a meeting, or some other sacrifice?

Fit: Are my skills and techniques able to address the client's problem? Is there something about the client that makes my type of treatment contraindicated? Does what I do fit what the client wants and is willing to engage in? Are they able to dependably travel to your location for appointments (or access virtual appointments)?

Fees: Can this client reasonably afford my regular rate? Can they afford enough sessions on a regular enough basis for the treatment to be effective? If they need a sliding scale or barter arrangement, is that something that I can afford to do? For how long? Will I be sustainable if I have to turn away a full-fee client because I have taken on this arrangement for this client? Will I resent this client if that happens?

Other considerations: What kind of rapport do I have with this client? Do I feel physically and emotionally safe with them? Is there anything about them or their problem that brings up strong emotional reactions in me that would make it difficult to work with them? Are there any dual relationships to consider? Are they in any of my communities, and, if so, how would them becoming my client affect our professional relationship as well as our individual experiences and comfort in that community?

14. A Love Note to My Fellow Helpers and Healers

I like to envision the whole world as a jigsaw puzzle ... If you look at the whole picture, it is overwhelming and terrifying, but if you work on your little part of the jigsaw and know that people all over the world are working on their little bits, that's what will give you hope.

-Jane Goodall

Dear fellow healers and helpers,

I hope you know how brave you are to have gotten this far. We spend so much time helping others and dispensing information that it takes a special humility and courage to take the time to admit to and learn how to manage our more tender spots.

Please be gentle with yourself as you move forward. The stumbling and slipping is all part of the learning.

Know your worth. Remember the value of your presence and energy, how even the smallest intervention you offer a client carries with it all those years of study and practice. Keep boundaries that allow you to use those resources intentionally rather than at the whim of others.

Make decisions with sustainability in mind. Sure, we signed up to help others. That doesn't mean that we signed away our right to make sure our own needs are met. We can only give all of ourselves for a short while, but we can give a mindfully chosen portion of ourselves for much, much longer.

Stay flexible and open to mystery. You may find opportunities to apply your skills that never existed before, that you can't imagine now.

And most of all, thank you. I don't know most of you, but I can picture you in your offices, standing by massage tables, listening on phones, flipping through reference books, writing progress notes, meeting with treatment teams, driving to sit by a bedside, washing your hands, squinting at schedules, gathering referrals, trying to make it all work. I can also sense the moments of doubt, overwhelm, worry, exhaustion, boredom, pain, and sadness.

So please, let yourself have a chance. You don't have to use everything in this book. I just ask that you try a handful of ideas to support yourself and the wonderful work you do. You, your clients, and the people in your life deserve it.

I wish you plenty of whatever you need most in the days to come. We are all with you.

Warmly,
Dr. Jo

Keys to Being a Sustainable Helper

1. You can't fix them--because they're not broken.

2. You're not going to have all the answers. Share what you know as truthfully as possible, seek guidance on what you don't know, and acknowledge that some mystery will always remain.

3. Being with can be as helpful as doing for, sometimes even more so.

4. You don't have to be perfect to be helpful, but you do have the responsibility to continually work to be aware of your biases, gaps in your expertise, and personal issues.

5. Listen more than you talk, especially when first meeting a client.

6. Think resilient rather than positive.

7. It's not yours to hold...let things flow through you.

8. You have more room than you think. You have space for everything you have and will experience.

9. You're never alone. You're surrounded by nature, supported by generations of past and present helpers.

10. Just as your clients grow and change, you and the ways you do your work are allowed to evolve over time.

15. Resources

15.1 Resources for Additional Support

Here are some hotline resources in case you or your client need something more than self-soothing:

National Suicide Prevention Lifeline: 1-800-273-8255 or chat online at https://suicidepreventionlifeline.org/

TransLifeline: 877-565-8860 https://www.translifeline.org/

Domestic Violence Hotline: 1-800-799-7233 or chat online at https://www.thehotline.org/help/

The Trevor Project (for LGBTQIA people under 25): 1-866-488-7386 or chat online at https://www.thetrevorproject.org/

Here's a link to a list of Warmlines for times when you might not be in a dangerous crisis but still really need to talk to someone: https://screening.mhanational.org/content/need-talk-someone-warmlines

Quarantine Chat is not a crisis line. It is a free project offering another way to connect with others https://quarantinechat.com/

15.2 Websites and Videos

Videos for the Self-Soothing Tips:

"Voo" Demonstration: https://youtu.be/MxiSUabkj24

iRest Yoga Nidra video: https://youtu.be/58WN8WqH1LM

Butterfly Hug: https://youtu.be/iGGJrqscvtU

Legs on a Chair:
http://www.notesfromahumbleyogini.co.uk/tag/spondylolisthesis/

Acceptance and Commitment Therapy:

Association for Contextual Behavioral Science
https://contextualscience.org/

Russ Harris https://www.actmindfully.com.au/

ACT Matrix trainers
https://www.theactmatrixacademy.com/certified-act-matrix-trainers-coaches

15.3 Other Books You Might Like

Big Magic: Creative Living Beyond Fear by Elizabeth Gilbert

Bright-Sided: How Positive Thinking Is Undermining America by Barbara Ehrenreich

Burnout: The Secret to Unlocking the Stress Cycle by Emily Nagoski & Amelia Nagoski

I Thought It Was Just Me (but it isn't): Making the Journey from "What Will People Think?" to "I Am Enough" by Brené Brown

It's OK That You're Not OK: Meeting Grief and Loss in a Culture That Doesn't Understand by Megan Devine

Letters to a Young Therapist by Mary Pipher

On Being a Therapist (Fifth Edition) by Jeffrey A. Kottler

Teaching Yoga: Exploring The Teacher Student Relationship by Donna Farhi

The Happiness Trap: Stop Struggling, Start Living by Russ Harris

The Needs of The Dying: A Guide for Bringing Hope, Comfort, and Love to Life's Final Chapter by David Kessler

The Places That Scare You: A Guide to Fearlessness in Difficult Times by Pema Chodron

The 10-Day Career Cleanse: Find Your Zen at Work by Lynn Chang

Training Your Dragon by Scott Baker

Trauma Stewardship: An Everyday Guide to Caring for Self while Caring for Others by Connie Burk and Laura van Dernoot Lipsky

Seven Thousand Ways to Listen: Staying Close to What is Sacred by Mark Nepo

Why Zebras Don't Get Ulcers: The Acclaimed Guide to Stress, Stress-Related Diseases, and Coping (Third Edition) by Robert M. Sapolsky

15.4 Podcasts and Online Courses

Magic Lessons with Elizabeth Gilbert (creativity and encouragement to use your gifts)

Abundant Practice Podcast with Allison Puryear (for therapists, but some episodes might be useful for other fields as well)

The Private Practice Startup with Dr. Kate Campbell and Katie Lemieux (for therapists)

The Practice of the Practice Podcast with Joe Sanok (for therapists)

The Money Sessions Podcast with Tiffany McLain. All about money fears and how to start charging what you're worth. Her Fun with Fees Calculator at https://www.heytiffany.com/ is an excellent tool for any service provider to use when setting or raising your fees.

Promote Yourself to CEO Podcast with Racheal Cook. Also highly recommend her free resources. https://rachealcook.com/

Empathy Rising: Side Hustles for Therapists in Private Practice with Marissa Lawton (lots of good marketing advice here as well)

Level Up Your Course Podcast with Janelle Allen (creating and marketing online courses)

The Creative Penn Podcast with Joanna Penn (writing and publishing) Between her podcast and her website, she offers just about everything you need to know to write and publish a book.

Podschool with Rachel Corbett (learning how to podcast) She has a free guide to starting podcasting on her website https://rachelcorbett.com.au/

15.5 References

Please note that these are by no means all of the articles on these topics, and research continues to evolve even as we speak. I offer them here as overviews and starting points for learning about these areas.

Abramowitz, J. S., Tolinb, D. F., & Street, G. P. (2001). Paradoxical effects of thought suppression: A meta-analysis of controlled studies. *Clinical Psychology Review, 21*(5), 683-703.

Cox, D. (2017, April 27). *The curse of the people who never feel pain.* BBC Future. https://www.bbc.com/future/article/20170426-the-people-who-never-feel-any-pain

Feijó, F. R., Gräf, D. D., Pearce, N., & Fassa, A. G. (2019). Risk factors for workplace bullying: A systematic review. *International Journal of Environmental Research and Public Health, 16*(11), 1945. https://doi.org/10.3390/ijerph16111945

Fessenden, M. (2015, January 2021). *This woman can't feel fear.* Smithsonian Magazine. https://www.smithsonianmag.com/smart-news/woman-cant-feel-fear-180953988/

Freeman, A., & Dolan, M. (2001). Revisiting Prochaska and DiClemente's stages of change theory: An expansion and specification to aid in treatment planning and outcome evaluation. *Cognitive and Behavioral Practice, 8*(3), 224-234. https://www.sciencedirect.com/science/article/abs/pii/S107 7722901800572

Merriam-Webster. (n.d.). *Sustainable.* https://www.merriam-webster.com/dictionary/sustainable

Nahum, D., Alfonso, C. A., & Sönmez, E. (2019). Common Factors in Psychotherapy. In: Javed A., Fountoulakis K. (eds) *Advances in Psychiatry.* Springer, Cham. https://doi.org/10.1007/978-3-319-70554-5_29

Rosanbalm, K. D., & Murray, D. W. (2017). *Caregiver Co-regulation Across Development: A Practice Brief.* OPRE Brief #2017-80. Washington, DC: Office of Planning, Research, and Evaluation, Administration for Children and Families, US. Department of Health and Human Services. http://dhss.alaska.gov/abada/ace-ak/Documents/Co-Regulation_Duke.pdf

Taylor, J. B. (2008). My stroke of insight: A brain scientist's personal journey. New York, NY: Viking Adult.

Prochaska and
  DiClemente, 28, 156
progressive muscle
  relaxation, 74
PTSD, 38, 75
public speaking, 121
pyramid schemes, 26
racism, 32, 114
rates, 23, 120
refer, 105
referrals, 145
resistant, 97
retraumatized, 17
romantic, 114
Russ Harris, 139
safety, 104
scarcity, 22, 24, 86
schedule, 22, 23, 76, 105,
  118, 120, 142, 145
schedules, 22, 23, 148
Self-betrayal, 23
Self-care, 23, 124
self-compassion, 101
Self-compassion, 127
senses, 84
services, 23, 24, 58, 99,
  106, 123
sexual, 114
sexuality, 115
shame, 14, 15, 35, 36, 38,
  43, 44, 45, 67, 98, 103,
  104, 105
Shame, 97
social justice, 33
socioeconomic status, 115
spirit animal, 33

stages of change, 28, 30
stakeholders, 142
stickers, 138
stress, 17, 21, 32, 70, 144
suicide, 6
supervisees, 115
sustainability, 17, 22, 148
sustainable, 8, 9, 47, 81,
  87, 100, 119, 120, 123,
  137, 145, 157
teacher trainings, 8, 10
telehealth, 123
termination, 29
Thomas Edison, 97
threatening, 104
tools, 5, 15, 24, 32, 38, 48,
  69, 70, 81, 95, 100, 101,
  103
trauma, 6, 7, 8, 16, 65, 67,
  75, 95, 121, 130
tribe, 33
triggered, 17, 75, 76, 77
unsolicited advice, 95
Urbach-Wieth disease, 80
validation, 98
Validation, 65
Vanessa Stone, 32, 96
vision quest, 33
Voo, 72, 152
white supremacy, 32
Willfulness, 90
Willingness, 89
WOE, 83, 85, 86, 88, 103
workshops, 121
Yoga Nidra, 74

Acknowledgements

I'm not sure how to even begin to list everyone who has helped make this book possible. I can start with the obvious: gratitude to Amrit Elise Mayton for another magical cover and realizing that morning glories would be the perfect was to represent the cycles of helping and healing. Many thanks to Joanna Penn, Orna Ross, and the Alliance of Independent Authors for teaching me everything I know about publishing and keeping me encouraged and inspired. A warm thank you and an even warmer big pot of stone soup to the Stillwater writer retreat group whose excitement when I read the intro aloud made it clear that this book needed to exist. To my multitude of teachers over the years, both living and via books: I hope I have passed along even a tiny percent of what I've learned from you. Endless gratitude to my family both here and on the other side, for cheering me on and keeping me laughing. The same gratitude extends to my furry family, tirelessly sleeping by my side while I typed. And, always, *merci beaucoup* to my partner Jack, for everything you are and do to help me be everything I can be.

And last, but not least, thanks to YOU for reading and for all the work you do in the world to help others!

This single-page printable full-color PDF poster of the *10 Keys to Being a Sustainable Helper* can serve as a reminder of your intentions to build a practice of being a sustainable helper & healer. Consider it a small token of thanks for all that you do for others—and for yourself!

You'll also receive occasional emails from me so you'll never miss out on future offerings and special subscriber-only promotions (you can unsubscribe anytime—I'll miss you, but I'll understand).

Here's the link to claim your free thank-you gift today:

https://bit.ly/theyrenotbroken

ALSO BY DR. JO ECKLER

I Can't Fix You—Because You're Not Broken: The Eight Keys to Freeing Yourself From Painful Thoughts and Feelings

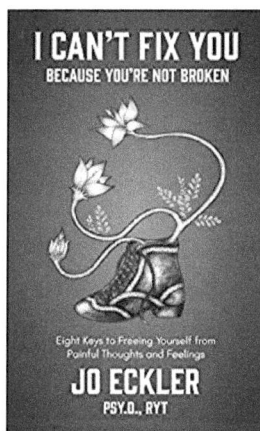

Available in e-book, paperback, hardcover, and audiobook anywhere you buy books, or ask your local library to add it to their collection.

Bulk discounts available for helpers and educators

Learn more at www.joeckler.com

Read on for a sample.

From *I Can't Fix You*: Of Toasters and Humans

You are not a toaster. At least, if you are reading this, I am assuming you're not a toaster. I know appliances are get-ting smarter every day with technology, but I'm guessing they're still a long way from picking up self-help books.

Now that we've established that you're (most likely) not a toaster, here's why that matters. You're not a toaster because you can't break. Appliances break, windows break, KitKat bars break, coffee breaks (wheee! Puns!), but people don't break.

"But Dr. Jo," you say. "I feel so broken! I feel damaged and shattered and deficient. I feel like there is something in-herently wrong with me, and if anyone ever found out what it was, they would despise me."

You feel how you feel—I will never argue about what emotions you may be experiencing at any given time. All emotions are valid. Even those that aren't attached to reality.

However, here's the deal. Although you may feel broken and like every cell in your body is screaming that it's true, you're not actually broken.

Read that through a few more times. That's right: you're not actually broken. You don't have to believe it yet, or ever. I just ask that you give me the rest of this book before you decide.

By the way, you might notice that I use "we" an awful lot in this book. I do that on purpose. I'm writing about common human experience, so it's likely that I've been there, that you've been there, and that your roommate who picks up this book when you leave it in the bathroom and their smartphone battery has died has been there. Hence, "we."

Because we're all in this, together.

CHAPTER ONE

From *I Can't Fix You*: Why We're Having This Conversation

Sometimes people look at the word "psychologist" in my title and decide that I have somehow bypassed pain, sorrow, and anxiety and have a completely put-together life. That my floors are spotless, my checkbook balanced, and my mind a sunshiny meadow swept by sweet breezes that smell faintly of lavender. This gets even worse when they see "yoga teacher" and they start adding on a perfectly balanced diet of dark leafy greens and sustainably harvested nuts between my hours of daily yoga and blissful meditation practice.

What a load of B.S. I can't speak for all mental health professionals and yoga teachers, but I came to this work—was pushed into this work—by life events that ambushed me, overwhelmed my emotional and mental defenses, and mugged me in dark alleys.

And oh, boy howdy did they take me down. Way down. Like making deals with myself that if things didn't improve in the next five years that I would kill myself down. I'll spare you the whole list. Suffice it to say that I renewed that deal with myself twice between the ages of 15 and 25. Things didn't get a whole lot easier after age 25, but I felt more able to hang in there.

I tried so many things to make those awful feelings go away. I poured alcohol, cigarettes, ice cream, and pizza into that emptiness inside, hoping to fill the void for even a moment. I tracked my thoughts. I recited affirmations. I walked. I listened to happy music. I tried to look on the bright side of life. I checked out armfuls of self-help books from the library. I got a degree. Then a doctorate. I moved to other cities, other states. I broke off romances, bounced into new beds. I binged on French films, on marathons of reality shows. I read The Bell Jar and Prozac Nation and cried in recognition (when I wasn't beating myself up for being so unhappy when I had so much going for me).

Gradually other things crept into my awareness, like the concept of mindfulness. I was lucky enough to be able to access training and books through my job as a psychologist that let me explore mindfulness, which was a gateway to yoga, which was a door to other forms of being present and sitting with the tough stuff that life kicks up.

Along with all of those things, I owe immense gratitude to Acceptance and Commitment Therapy, which has the fun acronym ACT (pronounced like the verb "to act"). I took a training about ACT right before one of my dear coworkers was killed in an automobile accident while on the way to work, and it gave me the tools to navigate through that and its aftermath without completely falling apart. I continue to lean on these principles day after day both personally and in my work with my clients. My offerings to you here are deeply infused with the principles of ACT, so if you like them, I encourage you to seek out a therapist trained in ACT or some of the other wonderful self-help books based in ACT. I owe immense gratitude to all who have worked to develop this therapy and who have trained me, especially Steven Hayes and Robyn Walsh. You can learn more and access a directory of ACT practitioners at https://contextualscience.org/

We're having this conversation because I know you've been suffering. I know that you're getting tired of trying everything you can to make the pain stop, striving to get to some kind of peace in your life. I know that it can feel so scary to be in the world when everyone else seems to have it together and yet the seemingly smallest thing can launch a panic at-tack or a flashback or a paralyzing barrage of self-loathing and shame. I know staying at home, staying in bed, staying small gets really boring—and yet to try anything else can feel terrifying. I know sometimes you lose hope, and sometimes you don't dare hope for fear of being disappointed.

Dear, dear one, please hang on a little longer. Read this book. Try it on. I can't make anything go away, but I want to offer you what I've found that has helped me and many others be able to take the steps to start living, not just dragging ourselves from hour to hour. It's not going to be quick and easy, but it'll be worth it.

Keep reading—visit www.joeckler.com or anywhere you buy books to get your copy today.

ABOUT THE AUTHOR

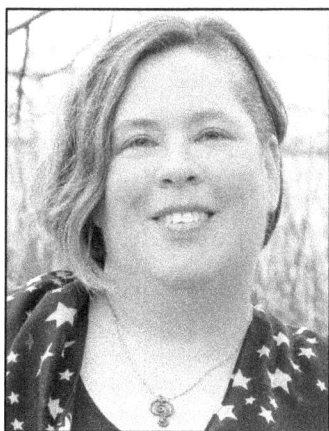

Dr. Jo Eckler is a licensed clinical psychologist and registered yoga teacher trained in energy work, sound healing, and as a death & mourning doula. The author of *I Can't Fix You— Because You're Not Broken: The Eight Keys to Freeing Yourself From Painful Thoughts and Feelings*, they've also appeared in numerous media outlets, including *O Magazine*, *Health*, *Bustle*, and *Huffington Post*. Their mission is to help others find more self-compassion, meaning, and conscious choice in their lives. Learn more at www.joeckler.com

ABOUT THE PUBLISHER

Spiral Staircase Publishing got its name from a strong belief that healing is like walking up a spiral staircase. Sometimes we get tired, sometimes it seems daunting, and sometimes we'd rather just sit for a while. We can feel like we're going in circles and getting nowhere. However, each time we circle around, we have moved up a little higher, we have learned a little more, and we have a little more breathing space from the initial hurt. Let's all keep walking, together, up towards the light. Wherever you are on your journey, we hope our books offer you encouragement humor, and support along the way.
www.spiralstaircasepublishing.com

www.ingramcontent.com/pod-product-compliance
Lightning Source LLC
Chamhershurg PA
CBHW060335030426
42336CB00011B/1353